TUNE IN TO
YOUR BABY

BECAUSE BABIES DON'T COME WITH AN INSTRUCTION MANUAL

RUTH OSHIKANLU

First published in Great Britain in 2012 by 90 Day Books, a trading name of Meaningful Goals Ltd., Sussex, England. www.90daybooks.com

Copyright © 2012 by Ruth Oshikanlu, all rights reserved.

Ruth Oshikanlu has asserted her right under the Copyright, Designs and Patents Act 1988 to be identified as the author of this work.

No part of this book may be used or reproduced, stored in a retrieval system, or transmitted in any form or any means, electronic, mechanical, photocopying, recording, scanning, or otherwise, except as permitted by the Copyright, Designs and Patents Act 1988, without either the prior written permission of the publisher or the author.

This book is sold subject to the condition that it shall not, by way of trade or otherwise, be lent, resold, hired out, or otherwise circulated without the publisher's prior consent in any form of binding or cover other than that in which it is published and without a similar condition, including this condition, being imposed on the subsequent purchaser.

Limit of Liability/Disclaimer of Warranty: While the publisher and author have used their best efforts in preparing this book, they make no representations or warranties with respect to the accuracy or completeness of the contents of this book and specifically disclaim any implied warranties of merchantability or fitness for a particular purpose. The advice and strategies contained herein may not be suitable for your situation. If in doubt, you are advised to consult a qualified medical practitioner. Neither the publisher nor author shall be liable for any loss of profit or any other commercial damages, including but not limited to special, incidental, consequential, or other damages.

Author's photograph by Slaine Montgomery.

Edited by Clare Christian and Kevin Bermingham.

Book interior design and typesetting by Pedernales Publishing, LLC.

Front cover design by Pedernales Publishing, LLC.

Diagrams by Ruth Oshikanlu.

British Library Cataloguing in Publication Data.

A catalogue record for this book is available from the British Library.

Paperback edition.
ISBN 978-1-908101-35-8

Praise for
Tune In To Your Baby
Because Babies Don't Come With An Instruction Manual
by Ruth Oshikanlu

'"Ruth has a unique perspective as a mother and health visitor which gives this book a perfect balance of personal experience, theory and genuinely practical advice on pregnancy through to parenting. As a new mother myself, this book lessened the feeling of parenthood being a journey into the unknown, and gave me insightful information to use in my life with my baby. The appendix, **My Baby Manual**, inspired me to keep challenging my own assumptions, and to take action rather than just read the book. I recommend the book to anyone thinking of having a baby, parents-to-be, and new parents.'
Joanne Caddy, mother of one

'I really enjoyed reading the book. It provides invaluable information about pregnancy, delivery and the difficult job of raising a child. It also tells the story of the writer's amazing journey into pregnancy and motherhood and how her life changed since the conception of Joshua. It celebrates the miracle of giving birth, as well as the joys and challenges this brings with it.'
Simona Bartocci, journalist and mother of two

'Ruth, I really enjoyed reading your book and sharing your experiences. I just wish I had read it years ago! It is so practical and reassuring. By sharing your learning it will make a huge difference to mothers of all ages and backgrounds. For me the message throughout "seeing things through your baby's eyes" comes across really clearly and is a useful tip. It made me realise that my time with my midwife was very much focused on the physical aspects and never covered any of these practical measures on how to cope. It was helpful thinking about the baby's delivery and experience of

birth and how it is so important to make those bonds early with skin-to-skin contact etc. The best thing is that you continue to deliver the same messages of being mindful throughout and for the reader your personal messages are really powerful.'
> Lucy Clement, district nurse and mother of two

'I thoroughly enjoyed Ruth's book. What I really like about the book is that it comes from the heart. It's a unique blend of a mum's perspective with lots of wise wisdom from a health professional who has years of experience and a wealth of knowledge to share. It is full of practical advice and information that is so crucial for new parents to know. Reading this book will help you form tighter bonds with your baby and make those first few months that are so tough emotionally and physically so much easier. I will be recommending this book to all new parents.'
> Helen Turier, ex-military nurse, successful businesswoman, author and mother of three

'Ruth, you have made this topic very easy to understand with clear and precise guidance for parents to follow. The style of your writing is one that can be used by a parent who may have limited education but does not patronise a parent who may have had a university education, which must be very difficult to achieve, as I am sure that parents from both educational extremes face the same dilemmas, anxiety and worries about being the best parent that they can be. It is gratifying to hear that even with all your experience, you too faced the same worries, which makes the book very empathic as you are able to offer reassurance both from the perspective of a mother and a health professional.'
> Maureen Major, learning disability nurse

Also by Ruth Oshikanlu

My Baby Manual: Because Babies Don't Come with An Instruction Manual.

(This A4-sized workbook replicates the appendix contained within *Tune In To Your Baby: Because Babies Don't Come With An Instruction Manual*)

This book is dedicated to my dad and mother – Nathan and Honey who have always been my rocks and taught me a lot of what I know as a parent. Also my brothers Nicholas and Michael who have supported me in parenting my son. And to my wonderful son Joshua who continues to teach me so much about how to parent and who brings out the best in me as I journey through parenthood.

'My personal vision is a world where every parent embraces and enjoys their role as parents despite its many challenges, meeting the needs of their child(ren) without sacrificing their needs.

I believe that most people want to parent well regardless of the situation that they find themselves in. I also am of the opinion that every parent is an expert in their circumstances.

My mission is to use my passion for empowering women to raise their babies and my proficiency in enabling them to find their solutions to enjoy being parents and succeed in parenting.

With some insight into why babies act the way they do, I believe that every parent can tune in to their baby, find out what they need, meet them and enjoy parenting.'

Ruth Oshikanlu, 2012

Contents

Acknowledgements xvii

Foreword xxi

Introduction 1

Chapter 1 – I Didn't Plan For This! 5

    Finding Out – "Oh no! I'm Pregnant!" 5

    Telling Others 6

    Change: Embrace It or Resist It – The Choice is Yours! 8

    Another Setback 9

    Can I Control It? 11

    Positive Thinking – The Science Behind It 12

    Manage Yourself 14

        Have a Backup Plan 14

        Mind 14

        Nutrition 15

        Exercise and Sleep 16

    Manage Your Expectations 17

    Yet Another Setback! 18

    Induction of Labour 19

    Labour and Delivery 20

    Neonatal Intensive Care Unit 23

    Breast-feeding 24

    Not Another Setback – I Can't Handle This! 24

    Sharing My Learning 26

Chapter 2 – Who Are You? – Getting To Know Your Baby ... 27

    Finding Out That You Are Pregnant 27

    Coming to Terms with Being Pregnant 28

    First Trimester 31

        Booking Appointment 32

The First Scan (Dating Scan) 33
The Second Trimester 34
    Baby's Brain Development in the Womb 34
    Connect With Your Baby 35
    Use It or Lose It! 36
    Twenty Week Scan 36
    What's In a Name? 37
    Communication – Look, Listen, and Feel 39
    Baby and Me Time 40
    Power of Touch 41
    Baby's First Kick 42
The Last Trimester 42
    Nesting 43
    Prepare for Motherhood 43
    Imagine Life With a Baby – Prepare to Enjoy It! 43
    Your Role as A Mother 44
    Some You Lose, Some You Gain! 44
    Prepare to Breastfeed Whilst Pregnant 45
    Preparing for Labour and Birth 46
    Antenatal Classes 47
    Birth Planning 47
Labour 50
    Pain Relief 50
    Medical Pain Relief 51
    Natural Methods of Pain Relief 51
    Mindset 52
    What if Things Don't go According to Plan? 54
    Prematurity 54
    Induction of Labour 55
    Instrumental Delivery – Forceps Delivery or Vacuum Extraction ... 55
    Caesarean Section 56

Problems After the Birth of Your Baby 57
    Sick Child 57
    Sick Mum 59
Sharing My Learning 61

Chapter 3 – I've Had the Baby, What Do I Do Next? 63

Labour and Birth Through Your Baby's Eyes 64
What a Hard Life! 67
Replicate the Womb Conditions for Baby Outside the Womb 68
Use Your Baby's Senses 70
Reading and Responding to Your Baby's Cues 72
Reading and Responding to Your Baby's States 73
    Deep Sleep 73
    Light Sleep 74
    Drowsy/Dozing 74
    Quiet Alert 74
    Active Alert 74
    Crying 75
Containment 76
Bonding and Attachment 77
Breast-feeding 78
Sleep 84
Understanding What Your Baby Needs 85
Love 89
Learning Through Play 89
I'm a Mum! 90
Motherhood: It's all Learning and Growing 92
Sharing My Learning 94

Chapter 4 – WOW! No One Said It Would Be This Hard 97

Practice Doesn't Make Perfect! 99
Parenting is Learning 100

Making Decisions? Remember, It's *Your* Baby!.........................103
Transactional Analysis..104
    Parent Ego State..104
    Adult Ego State..105
    Child Ego State..105
Making Decisions as a Parent – Be Adult About It!...................106
Your Baby is Unique – Don't Compare!.....................................107
Be Patient! View Each Day as a Learning Experience...............107
Feeding..108
Crying...109
Sleeping...110
You are Your Baby's Teacher!..112
Get Organised!..113
    Manage Your Time..113
    Pareto Principle (The 80:20 Rule)............................114
    Plan Your Day, Daily!...115
Be Balanced..116
Trust That Things Will Eventually Fall Into Place......................117
When Things Don't Go to Plan...118
    Loneliness..119
    Postnatal Depression..119
    Domestic Abuse..121
    Relationship Breakdown – Single Parenting...........122
Don't Become a Victim...123
Not Yet! No Such Thing as Failure!..125
Going Back to Work...126
Guilt – Use It or Lose It!...127
Work/Life Balance..129
Continue Loving, Playing and Learning with Your Baby............131
Sharing My Learning..133

Chapter 5 – Help, My Child Has Mutated! The Toddler Years......... 135

What are the Toddler Years? 136
Fussy Eating – Why it Happens 138
How to Manage Fussy Eating 138
Sleeping Problems – Why They Happen 141
How to Manage Sleeping Problems 143
Tantrums – Why They Happen 145
How to Manage Tantrums 147
Potty Training 151
Communicate With Your Toddler 153
Promoting Speech 154
There's No Point Saying 'No!'... 157
What Kind of Parent Are You?.. 159
    Authoritarian Parent – high control, low acceptance and nurture 159
    Permissive Parent – low control, high acceptance and nurture 159
    Passive Parent – low control, low acceptance and nurture 160
    Authoritative Parent – high control, high acceptance and nurture 160
Managing Toddler Behaviour.. 161
Love and Manage Yourself... 162
Love Your Toddler.. 163
Sharing My Learning 165

Chapter 6 – Putting It All Into Practice 167

Important Notice 171

Bibliography and References 173

Online References and Useful Websites 179

About The Author 183

Appendix – My Baby Manual 185

Acknowledgements

I would like to thank the following people who supported me through the journey of creating this book and enabled me to achieve my goal of becoming an author.

Firstly my parents Nathan and Honey and my brothers Nicholas and Michael who were excellent sources of support and childcare whilst writing the book. You have always had an incredible belief in me. As such, I can't give up on me when the going gets tough, because you never have.

Thank you very much Joshua, for teaching me how to parent you. It was because of the experiences I went through whilst having you that brought about the birth of this book. I feel very honoured to be your mother and am ever so grateful to you for teaching me how to love unconditionally.

I'd like to thank Kevin Bermingham, my publisher and 'author's mentor'. Without his step-by-step 90-day book writing programme, this book would not have been born in such a short period of time. You have definitely increased my belief that I can do anything I'm committed to. Not only have I learned to be disciplined, but also how to enjoy the art of writing a book despite the intensity of the programme. I remember feeling quite overwhelmed after planning my book. But with your support, I gave birth to my first book and have a hunger for writing many more.

I'm also very grateful to Johnson, Joshua's dad for assisting me in parenting our son, Joshua. The help you continue to provide always proves invaluable. Even though I'm single, I never feel alone in making informed choices for Joshua.

RUTH OSHIKANLU

A huge thank you as well, to Professor Dame Donna Kinnair who wrote the foreword for this book and who gives me continued support as a professional mentor.

I also want to express my profound gratitude for my book reviewers. Firstly, the lovely mums who took time out of parenting their infants to provide me with excellent feedback: Joanne Caddy, Helen Tarbuck, Simona Bartocci, Jackie Ng and Ekaterina Sazhina, and the professionals who despite their busy schedules made time to review the book's contents: Helen Turier, Yvonne Batson-Wright, Lucy Clement, Jane Cook, Maureen Major, Michelle Racey, Fawn Bess-Leith, Margaret Khumalo, Maggie Fisher and Bernadette Kinsella. Thanks for sharing my book writing journey with me and for the excellent feedback too.

I'd like to thank Dave Dawes and Agnes Fanning who are trainers and coaches on the *Nurse First* programme for facilitating my growth in confidence. I'm also grateful to Sandra Bennett for her role in writing this book. It was whilst on this programme the idea for the book developed. On one of the residential evenings, while in conversation with her about childbirth, I realised how much I have learned and grown as a parent. It was this conversation that ignited my intense desire to pen *Tune In To Your Baby*.

Many thanks also to Sonia White and Bukky Adeyemo for the incredible patience and generous support you gave me whilst editing this book. I'd also like to express my gratitude to my fabulous friends and colleagues – Cynthia Appiah, Gillian Lesforis, Jennifer Wilson, Kelley Webb-Martin, Sonia Stewart and Sonia White for being wonderful role models and enabling my professional growth.

I'd also like to thank everyone that has supported me on my journey – mentors, coaches, role models, friends and clients who have influenced my thinking and behaviour and facilitated my growth and development.

Most of all, I'd like to thank my Creator, the Almighty for supporting me during my difficult pregnancy and childbirth and continuing to allow me to learn to love and live whilst parenting my son Joshua.

Foreword

Reading this book has made me chuckle in so many places as Ruth describes the exceptional journey of motherhood. She transports the reader using aspects of her own personal journey to guide you from the time you find out you are pregnant, using key milestones in your baby's development from conception through to early toddlerhood. This book provides parents with the necessary information and knowhow to understand their baby's needs and feelings; so that they have the tools to support the rearing of an individual with its own thoughts and desires. Ruth explores many of the thoughts and feelings that this unique experience throws up for women and their partners. She provides practical ways to cope with the journey, and explores the medical and sociological theories that underpin child development and parenting. Ruth tackles with professional expertise, both as a mother, midwife and health visitor, the difficulties we experience in the everyday challenges that life throws at us during this period and helps us understand how much good planning and a positive focus can help in overcoming these difficulties. This book attempts to coach the reader through a time when self-analysis, forward planning and reflection will prove more helpful than any prescription.

Professor Dame Donna Kinnair

Introduction

Dear reader, many thanks for your investment in this book. In it I share my pregnancy journey right through until my son was about four years old. My name is Ruth and my son is called Joshua. 2004 was a very difficult year for me, but it was then that I learned the most vital lessons in my life. Finding out I was pregnant right through to having a baby and becoming a single parent was the most difficult time of my life so far. The feelings of total powerlessness that overcame me as I tried to grow my baby whilst trying to remain sane still bring tears to my eyes. What further compounded my story is that I was a midwife when I had this experience. So I understood what was happening to me. However, I didn't know how to handle the experiences. Since then I have become a health visitor and a life coach. Looking back I have learned so much personally and professionally. As I acquired new knowledge, I often said to myself, 'I wish I knew that when I needed it!' Hence one reason for writing this book.

Another reason for writing this book is the emerging evidence about the importance of the care the baby receives in pregnancy through to the first two years of life. Advances in neuroscience have shown that there is a big relationship between early brain development and outcomes later in life, highlighting the fact that what a mum does in pregnancy and the first two years of life are crucial. A baby's brain develops in response to what he experiences at this time. As such, it is essential to ensure that a child's environment and experience – both in the womb and outside it are pleasurable as it is at this time the foundation blocks are laid. Thus, love will be stressed as a vital ingredient throughout this book – love for self and baby.

Parents often struggle to cope with the changes their new role brings and provide the care their infant needs. This can be especially difficult for first-time parents as the information contained in books, magazines and the Internet and offered by family and friends and even professionals often conflict with each other causing confusion. The pressure to get things right further compounds the problem, creating anxiety for parents and thus the baby. Hence another reason for writing this book. In my working life as a health visitor I continue to meet parents that are very anxious about what to do with their baby. They worry about doing the 'right' things and are sometimes confused because the professionals that they meet give them conflicting advice. They worry about the normal things that the baby does and think a baby crying is a reflection of how they are parenting.

This book is not a comprehensive manual, neither is it detailed in its content and will not cover all aspect of pregnancy, childbirth and parenting. However, it will highlight some key moments during pregnancy and the first four years of life that can impact on the mum's feelings and hence the development of the baby. The focus will be on the mum and baby, because she carries the baby in pregnancy and is often the main caregiver in the postnatal period. In it I will share my experiences in pregnancy, childbirth and raising my son Joshua. I will share how I coped with a very difficult pregnancy; what I learned from it; what I wished I had known at the time and what I have learned professionally from working as a nurse, midwife, health visitor, coach and most especially as a single parent. To prevent confusion, I will use the male pronoun when referring to the baby to make it easier distinguish between the mum and the baby.

As every baby and parent is unique I often do not utilise a *one size fits all* approach in my practise and as such will not be doing so in this book. The book aims to share some of the insights gained to assist you in finding your own solutions. It is not prescriptive in its approach as I believe we are all expert in our circumstances and with some knowledge, can generate our own solutions to any problems we may encounter. Instead I will share a range of suggestions and ask you a lot of questions with a view to you creating your own solutions. At the end of each chapter I will share my learning in the form of tips for success.

Chapter 1 will focus on my experiences in pregnancy and labour and the eventual birth of my son and how I coped. Chapter 2 will focus on normal pregnancy and concentrate on the baby's perspective: how you can get to know your baby and start to form a relationship with him. Helping your baby adapt to life outside the womb will be the focal point of Chapter 3. Chapter 4 will burst the myth of perfect parenting with suggestions on how to be content with being a *good enough* parent, whilst Chapter 5 will focus on toddlerhood. A final chapter gives tips on how to put it all into practice. The chapter titles were created from expressions I made whilst pregnant or as a parent. They are also synonymous with what I have heard other parents relate to me in my practice as a midwife and health visitor.

Babies do not come with an instruction manual. Therefore, I urge you to create your own.

The appendix of this book contains a toolkit to help you create your own baby manual. Alternatively, you may wish to purchase the A4-sized baby manual that I have written to accompany this book – *My Baby Manual: Because Babies Don't Come with An Instruction Manual.*

As you read through this book, you will be directed to the appendix to help you to complete your own baby manual. Look out for this symbol:

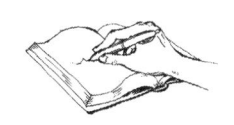

RUTH OSHIKANLU

*'The discipline of writing something down is
the first step to make it happen.'*
Lee Iacocca, Engineer and businessman

Let me start by telling you my story.

Chapter 1
I Didn't Plan For This

I can't remember the number of times I said this phrase in pregnancy, labour and after Joshua was born. Hence the reason for the title of this chapter.

Finding Out – "Oh no! I'm Pregnant!"

It all started on 10th March 2004 when I missed my period. The first feeling was that of denial. 'It can't be true,' I said to myself several times. I took the morning after pill as instructed within 72 hours four weeks earlier, so what was going on? My periods are very regular, but I thought maybe on this occasion it will be a few days late. So I waited but it never came. As if not finding out would change the result I waited a few days before testing. On my way to work three days after my expected period, I purchased a pregnancy kit and the two tests were as positive as they could be – thick blue lines. Still not convinced or rather in total denial, I purchased a more sophisticated testing kit that spells out the result. The result read PREGNANT. Every time I blinked I hoped to see the word NOT appear but it didn't show up and neither did my period come. In fact I had to wait over two years before I saw it again. My heart sank. This is not how I planned it! I thought. Not now! I said to myself. I'm not ready; this is bad timing… and so on.

Three months earlier, I had turned 30 and was working on night duty as a midwife. I remember feeling quite low in mood, regretting all that I had planned to achieve by 30 but not attained – no master's degree, no house of my own, no husband, no baby and even working nights – I thought I'd have given that up by now too. Little did I know that my life as I knew it would change dramatically. They say be careful what you wish for. Well I have learnt that the hard way!

All of a sudden the life I resented a few months before looked so appealing. However, being a natural problem solver I thought, this baby is here to stay, so I need to work around baby. Thoughts whirled round my head. I need an action plan. I am going to continue with the pregnancy but finish everything I'm currently doing more quickly. I need a new house. I need to finish the course I've just started. I need to leave my job as night shifts are not conducive to raising a baby. I've not even told my partner – he'll have to marry me before baby is born. And my family – where do I start? Being my father's only daughter, he's always dreamed about walking me down the aisle. Overwhelmed, I felt like disappearing. I closed my eyes several times, but it didn't happen. Despite being 30, I felt like a teenager. And that is how Joshua's journey to the world began.

Telling Others

Before I could tell anyone, I had to decide what I wanted. I was definitely continuing with the pregnancy so I wrote the list of everyone I would tell in order of priority. I had to tell Joshua's father first and although the pregnancy was unexpected he promised to support me whatever I decided. Next I told my brothers as I felt they would support me and assist me in telling my parents. They were shocked at first but very supportive. In order to tell my mother, I had to book a weekend break away in Paris and when I eventually told her, her first question was,

'Who is he?' Then she continued, 'You've got to get married!' and then, 'And before baby is born!' 'OK Mum,' I said. I had kind of guessed that. Then she said: 'Now how are we going to tell your dad?' Million dollar question I thought to myself, I definitely didn't want to be responsible for his death!

We both planned how we would tell my dad the news but what compounded the problem was having to tell him over the phone as my father lived in Nigeria at the time. I remember calling him a few days later and because of the tone of my voice he was close to tears thinking someone had died. I told him that it was worse than that as I felt I had totally disappointed him, knowing about his dream to walk me down the aisle. Once I told him he sobbed. 'You have gone and put the cart before the horse,' he said. 'But you'll always be my daughter and I still love you.' Even though he was in tears, I still felt his love. He asked what I was going to do. I told him I didn't know but that I was keeping the baby.

You may wonder what all the fuss was about. But I do strongly believe in children being raised by married parents having been raised that way myself. I felt a total failure as this was not how I had planned my life.

> *'We change our behaviour when the pain of staying the same becomes greater than the pain of changing. Consequences give us the pain that motivates us to change.'*
>
> Henry Cloud, Psychologist, leadership consultant and author

Change: Embrace It or Resist It – The Choice is Yours!

Change is defined in the dictionary as 'a passing from one phase to another,' (Collins English Dictionary, 2009). If only it were that simple. Change is difficult because it pushes us out of our comfort zone. The tendency is to fear or resist it especially if we cannot guarantee the outcome. Change can leave us in a state of paralysis if it is unexpected as it did in my case. It is uncomfortable, as it disrupts our control over outcomes. However, resisting change can have a ripping effect on those who won't let go. It induces worry, anxiety and frustration and can lead to depression. As such it is better to embrace it no matter how difficult it may seem.

Change is a fact of life and is vital for growth and life. It can be likened to a muscle that hurts when it is continuously flexed but over time becomes stronger and looks well defined. Brian Mayne, a mentor of mine, likened change to the wind that blows. We can't stop it and neither can we control it. Without wind a boat will be marooned in the middle of the sea. But the stronger the wind blows the more power you have to move towards your chosen destination. Instead of fighting the wind, we can set our sails in order to steer our boat in the direction we want. Thus, if we can change before we are forced to, it is a less painful experience. Once we decide to change in our hearts, it is evident in our actions. For a while I resisted change, wasting my time looking back at how my life could have been, but I made a conscious decision to embrace my new life and there was only one direction to move in – towards the future. And so I decided to face the music and plan my future with a child. Upon embracing change, I learned from it. I grew in strength and confidence and became the best person I could be. As a quote I once read states: 'change is like driving in a fog – you can't see very far, but you can make the whole trip that way,' (Edgar Lawrence Doctorow, Author).

Looking back I have successfully driven through the fog and boy, have I grown.

Another Setback

Between March and July, I tried to fast-track everything. I applied for a new job and got it. I completed the course I was doing and started planning the wedding as I had to get married before baby was born. I even managed to find a new home and planned to move into it by August but it all went pear-shaped at 21 weeks when I had my scan. On 21st July 2004, I went to work in the morning and left at lunchtime for my scan in the afternoon. During the scan everything was fine until the sonographer (the person performing the scan) asked rhetorically, 'where is the other leg?' I looked at the screen with dilated pupils thinking she'd better find the other leg and she certainly did. It was in the cervix (the neck of the womb) and my baby was on his way out. She said you'll have to go to theatre because your cervix is shortening. Of course I knew the score – as a midwife I had supported several women in this state, but I sure did not plan for this. Over the next few hours as I was prepared for theatre I was in total denial. 'I'm going to work tomorrow,' I kept saying to anyone who would listen. I saw several professionals – obstetricians, anaesthetists and midwives who informed me that I had to have a cervical stitch to hold the cervix closed as it was beginning to open up. I was informed several times about the risks associated with this procedure – accidental rupture of the membranes. If this happened, they would not be able to put the stitch in and if baby was born, they would just have to watch him die as he was under 24 weeks gestation. As they informed me about this I had to consent for the procedure and they kept checking my understanding as my face must have said it all: utter confusion: how did this happen? Why me? Why now?

I eventually had the stitch put in and thankfully the membranes were intact, but the cervix was so short they could only put a low stitch in and could not guarantee it would hold. During the night I prayed so hard and was overcome with guilt. Maybe if I had wanted this baby more, this would not have happened to me. I also felt guilty about taking the morning after pill. I thought it served me right. This is your punishment, I told myself continuously. Up until then, I was terrified that baby may not develop properly because I had taken emergency contraception. I remembered all the women I had looked after with this condition and I felt so sorry for myself because I knew I may have to spend the rest of my pregnancy in hospital. I was terrified, as some of the women I had looked after ended up losing their babies. I did not sleep a wink all night. I cried right through. I felt so alone. As the tears rolled down my cheeks, I felt a flutter in my belly. It was my baby! This was the first time I had sat still enough to feel him. I started to apologise to him telling him how much I loved him and how he meant the world to me. I told him that if he came out we'd all have to watch him die. I pleaded with him to stay inside me as this was the best place for him. The week before, his dad and I had argued about names. We agreed on a girl's name but could not decide on a boy's name. I wanted him to be called Jonathan (The Lord has given) and his dad wanted Joshua. As I had found out that I was having a boy during the scan, I instantly decided on Joshua because of its meaning – 'The Lord is salvation'. My baby had to be saved! I was not going to lose him! I started to use his name in our daily conversations and rubbed my belly every time he moved. I talked to him every day thanking him for staying an extra day. Little did I know that there was evidence behind what I was doing.

> *'Turn your wounds into wisdom.'*
> Oprah Winfrey, Media proprietor, talk show host, actress, producer, and philanthropist

Can I Control It?

After having the stitch put in, I had to have weekly cervical scans (scans of the cervix) in the Prematurity Clinic. Every time I attended the cervix had become shorter and I was so disappointed. I couldn't understand why. I was on continuous bed rest and had my legs elevated most of the day. I had my head down and legs elevated in the belief that in this position I could counter the effects of gravity pulling baby on the cervix. I only got up to go to the toilet. I asked to be put into a side room as being in a room where other women were going into labour caused me a lot of despair. By 24 weeks when I had the third weekly cervical scan, my cervix had shortened form 15mm to 5mm. My cervix was just 5mm from opening up! I was downhearted and cried all night. I pleaded with Joshua not to come out. That night I was given the first of two steroid injections. This was to mature his lungs, just in case he was born early. I told him that although I had been given the steroids, if he was born then, he would have to be ventilated and have tubes and needles in every orifice in his body. I kept telling him that it would be a very painful experience for both of us.

    That night passed and Joshua didn't come out and in that moment I decided I was going to regain some control. The news of my shortening cervix was not helping me. Sometimes ignorance is bliss. Whatever will be, will be: I told myself. Knowing would make no difference. I told the obstetrician at the Prematurity Clinic that I wouldn't be attending her appointments anymore. I was disappointed with her reaction as she thought I was in denial. Maybe I was. However, I believed that the procedure which involved inserting a probe into the vagina to view the cervix was not helping my condition because it was invasive in nature. More importantly, knowing the condition of my cervix was taking away my hope, which I felt was a powerful medicine that the medics were not prescribing.

I decided to start thinking positively. Normally, I am an optimist, but my situation had changed me greatly and it was so difficult to remain positive. I had made some friends in hospital who had the same condition and they were a great strength during this time as they would come in immediately after my scan and try to uplift me as I was crying. Unfortunately, one of them who was a few weeks ahead of me in her pregnancy had her baby at 25 weeks. Little did I know how this would affect me.

On 18th August 2004, I woke up at 5.00 a.m. and was convinced that my waters had gone. I pulled the emergency cord and screamed for the midwife. The midwife attended and I was screaming hysterically that my waters had broken. She checked my bed and it was completed dry. Even though the bed was completely dry, I felt it was wet and was completely distraught that she wouldn't believe me. It took three midwives to convince me that my bed was dry. I felt I was losing my mind! If only I knew then what I know now.

> 'You always do what you want to do. This is true with every act. Whatever you do, you do by choice. Only you have the power to choose for yourself.'
>
> W. Clement Stone, Businessman, philanthropist and author

Positive Thinking – The Science Behind It

Inside our heads we have about a hundred billion neurons (brain or nerve cells). Each one has arms called dendrites. Each dendrite is separated by a slight gap called a synapse. Whenever you have a thought, an impulse is sparked to make a connection with another arm so that the thought can spread, forming a pattern of understanding – a train of thought.

When the thought is positive, the positive impulse triggers the release of serotonin – a chemical that gives a feeling of happiness and wellbeing. This hormone also acts as a conductor that bridges the synaptic gap and allows your thought to flow freely and continue its journey. However, when the thought is negative, the release of cortisone is triggered. It gives you the feeling of sadness and depression and works like an insulator, blocking and limiting the free flow of thoughts. Cortisone is also one of the main hormones released by the adrenal gland in response to stress, a by-product of which is cortisol. Cortisol, along with adrenalin, elevates blood pressure and prepares the body for a fight or flight response.

Negative thinking can lead to stress which when experienced in pregnancy over a prolonged period can affect a woman's unborn baby as early as 17 weeks after conception, with potentially harmful effects on brain and development. Cortisol can affect the mum's vascular function, thereby reducing blood flow to the foetus, which could affect growth by reducing the amount of oxygen and nutrients that are delivered. The higher the level of cortisol in the mum's blood, the greater the level of cortisol in the amniotic fluid. Thus, the importance of positive thinking, especially in pregnancy cannot be over emphasised.

Despite knowing the above, it is very difficult to change a pattern of negative thinking once established. I had to start by asking myself what was good about my situation and what I could learn from it. Even though I felt helpless, there was so much to be grateful for. I got a journal and made a list of all the things I was grateful for with a goal to add one more thing each day. The things in my list included being in the Western world in a hospital that was advanced in technology to help me. The doctors were on my side even though it often didn't feel like it as I desperately wanted to go home. They had my best interests at heart – the safety of my baby. Joshua's dad was supportive and visited every day with cooked food.

My family was supportive and even though my father was thousands of miles away, he called every day to assure me of his love. Each day I would read the list out to affirm it to myself and for Joshua to hear. I would also pray every day asking God to give me strength especially when I felt low. Over time I grew in strength and learned resilience. Every day I remained pregnant was one more day for Joshua.

Manage Yourself

Have a Backup Plan

We all know it's important to have a backup plan, or Plan B but it's not always easy. When unplanned change hits us we can be taken aback. Almost like a bee hitting a glass window headfirst. It is destabilising. Once this happens it is worthwhile to regroup. Think about your original plan and ask yourself why it's not working. It must be noted that we can't always control what happens to us, but from my experience, one thing we do have control over is our thoughts.

Mind

The greatest learning for me is that we can't always control our circumstances but we can indeed control our reactions to any event we face and hence, the outcome. Wasting time over things we cannot control saps our energy and causes us undue anxiety and stress. It is better to endeavour to influence our circumstances. However, there are times when we can do neither. We then have to accept it. I decided to accept that I was not going home anytime soon and that the hospital was going to be my home for a very long time. I also accepted that I would be on my back for a long time, but would hopefully have a healthy baby to show for it. I planned my house move from my hospital bed and got my brothers and Joshua's dad to help me move. Fortunately most of my stuff had been packed in boxes prior to my hospital admission. But I had to trust that they would do it as best they could even if it may not have been to my entire satisfaction as I am a perfectionist and often a control freak.

Nutrition

In pregnancy it is essential for your baby to eat a healthy, well-balanced diet. A well-balanced diet is one that includes foods from all the food groups in appropriate amounts to ensure proper nutrition. Good nutrition ensures that all essential nutrients – carbohydrates, fats, protein, vitamins, minerals and water are supplied to the body and the baby to maintain optimal health and wellbeing. It is essential for normal organ development and functioning, especially the brain; growth and maintenance; resistance to infection and disease; and the ability to repair bodily damage or injury.

Knowing this, I had a huge problem with the hospital food. They rotated the food every two weeks and after two weeks of being an in-patient I lost my appetite for hospital food. When I had a growth scan and was told my baby was not growing well. I asked what they expected when I was living on hospital food? Even prisoners get better food, I retorted. I got my family to bring me food and they did every day until my food went missing from the communal fridge on the ward. I made everyone's life on the ward a misery and persuaded the staff to allow me to get a fridge and a microwave to give me some independence. They agreed as long as it was checked to be safe by the hospital's electrical department. I got my family to buy a small fridge to keep my food fresh and a microwave to warm my food and this afforded me some independence and kept the ward staff sane. After a month in hospital the television viewing fees were over a hundred pounds and resulted in my continuously moaning to the ward management. I was allowed to bring my laptop in and purchased a TV card to enable me to watch TV on it. Music was also a source of inspiration and I played music regularly to lift my moods when I was feeling down. Joshua also enjoyed listening to music and before long I could I determine the kind of music he liked. I enjoyed watching him move to the music I played.

Exercise and Sleep

Exercise in pregnancy has many benefits. It helps you sleep better, boosts your energy, reduces pregnancy discomfort, reduces stress, lifts your spirits and helps you prepare for labour and childbirth. Your body goes through an exhausting journey as it is creating a life and it is therefore important to get enough sleep in pregnancy to give your baby the best chance possible for being healthy. There is evidence that the amount of sleep you get in pregnancy can greatly influence the amount of time you spend in labour. The fewer the number of hours of sleep in pregnancy, the longer the length of labour, with women who get fewer than five hours of sleep a night having a greater chance of having a Caesarean section delivery.

I couldn't exercise as I was flat on my back, but I did leg exercises to prevent blood clots and thrombosis and arm exercises with the hanging bed frame. I committed to sleeping better as it would benefit me and my baby. And I did! The power of the mind is amazing. As I worried less I slept better and felt better. Hours became days. Days became weeks. Weeks became months, and I remained pregnant. At 28 weeks, on medical advice I decided to have another cervical scan. Was I amazed to find that my cervix had lengthened? It measured 15mm at 21 weeks, 5mm at 24 weeks and at 28 weeks – 35mm. The normal cervix measures 30 – 50mm. Mine was within normal range. I couldn't believe it! Looking back, I believe that I must have been under such immense stress that my baby was swimming in so much cortisol that he wanted to flee that environment. Once I relaxed, and embraced my state and managed my mind, my body healed itself and became an environment that was conducive for the baby to thrive.

Manage Your Expectations

I managed my expectations by taking one day at a time. I prepared my mind for the worst and hoped for the best. I celebrated every day I remained pregnant and praised Joshua for working with me. I told him how much I loved him and my plans for him. I read my journal to him every day and enjoyed listening to music with him. He often responded to music and I tried to read his reaction to it. I was beginning to enjoy my pregnancy. I started to work with the obstetricians instead of resisting them, getting as much information as I could from them but consciously choosing whatever advice served me and immediately dismissing any that didn't.

> *'Our greatest battles are those with our minds.'*
> Jameson Frank, Artist

Yet Another Setback!

At 29 weeks I was told by one of the consultants that I could go home. I was really excited and made plans. However, at the ward round another consultant advised me to wait another two weeks, as the chances were better if baby was born at 31 weeks. I was disappointed but understood the rationale behind the decision especially as I previously worked in a neonatal intensive care unit (NICU) and had looked after premature babies. The longer my baby stayed in my womb, the better the chances of survival outside it. I decided to heed the advice as I wanted the best chance for my baby. Nonetheless, the two weeks felt like two years. I decided to count down to the discharge date rather than up from the date the decision was made in order to give me a feeling of progression. Eventually 14 days passed and on that morning I decided to set the tone of the day. I got up early, got dressed to go home and packed all my bags. I sat on the bed eagerly waiting for the ward round so that I could go home. Eventually the doctors came and told me I could go home. I was elated! They suggested that I have a blood test before going home. Waiting for the blood test felt like forever. In time the phlebotomist came and took several bottles of blood. He told me that he would send them urgently and should get the results in a couple of hours. The midwife advised me to wait for the results as they also had to wait for my medication to be delivered from the pharmacy. After waiting about three hours the midwife finally came with my medication but the look on her face said it all. She informed me that the blood results were not good and I would need to be reviewed by the registrar. My heart sank. Surely it can't get any worse, I thought.

The registrar eventually came and gave me the bombshell. I had pre-eclampsia (a medical condition in which a pregnant woman develops high blood pressure, protein in the urine, unusual swelling of the hands, feet or face) and could not go home. I sobbed so much. I spent most of the day crying as I unpacked my bags. Over the next few days I had many investigations and was started on anti-hypertensives as my blood pressure spiralled out of control. Within a couple of weeks I was on four different blood pressure tablets and had to move out of my room onto the main ward as I needed to be monitored closely. I was also having blood tests three times a day to monitor my liver and kidney function. Within four weeks I had become so swollen the phlebotomist was having difficulty taking blood from my veins. On the 19th November, despite trying several times, the phlebotomist was unable to draw bloods. At the ward round the consultant obstetrician advised that I get a central line inserted into one of the big veins in my neck so they could get bloods to monitor the pre-eclampsia. I refused. I had had enough. So I agreed to have labour induced. As baby was still premature (36 weeks) I was advised to have the cervical stitch out and to be as active as I could in labour as baby would be unable to undergo a long labour. I agreed. In the week prior to Joshua's birth he was not as active as he usually was. Whenever, I informed the midwives and medics I was told it was because of the blood pressure medication that made me very drowsy. Thankfully in that period, I slept for most of the day and was not awake to worry. I felt reassured during the twice daily foetal monitoring as it was lovely to hear Joshua's heart beating and watching him play 'hide and seek' with the cardiotocograph (unborn baby's heart rate monitor).

Induction of Labour

The induction process began. I was moved to the labour ward and the cervical stitch was taken out. I cried so much because of the intense pain. When the stitch was inserted, it was done under a spinal block so I felt no pain. But when it was taken out, all I had was gas and air. The pain was so intense the tears just rolled from my eyes. I couldn't even scream. I felt so weak with pain that I pleaded with the obstetrician to take me to theatre to have a Caesarean section. The midwife that was with her reminded me that I wanted a normal delivery. Of course I wanted a normal delivery! But I was not mentally or physically prepared for the pain that I experienced when the stitch was removed. As a midwife, I had observed the procedure done several times, but the pain took me aback. I still feel it as I write.

Once the stitch was out, the prostaglandin gel to induce labour was applied and I was advised to mobilise, mobilise, mobilise. Desperate for a normal delivery, I walked all over the labour ward and the tranquillity room designed for labouring women to relax and keep mobile. I only sat down when I wanted to use the toilet. I had to have a vaginal examination every four hours to monitor my progress. My cervix was dilating to plan and every time the baby's heart rate was monitored he was coping with labour. At about 7.00 p.m. the contractions started but they were bearable. At about 8.00 p.m. the waters broke and I felt like pushing. I was excited as it looked like I was going to have a normal delivery.

> 'The greatest discovery of all time is that a person can change his future by merely changing his attitude.'
> Oprah Winfrey, Media proprietor, talk show host, actress, producer, and philanthropist

Labour and Delivery

I was moved to a labour room and introduced to a lovely midwife who was going to be responsible for my care. She did an internal examination and I was three centimetres dilated. I planned to have my baby delivered in eight hours and set my mind to endure for that length of time hoping to dilate a centimetre an hour. I walked around the room as much as I could. Joshua's dad was so supportive even though he could not say anything without getting a negative reaction from me. My cousin who was in her early twenties was also a rock and I was more tolerant of her. I laboured for the next eight hours and I had another internal examination hoping that I would almost be fully dilated. But I had only dilated an extra centimetre. I was distraught. The pain was intense and I was not coping. I asked for an epidural as the gas and air was not touching the pain.

It took an hour for the anaesthetist to attend but it felt like forever. I tried several positions short of standing on my head, but nothing seemed to help. I tried water, the floor, the ball, nothing helped. It was such a frightening experience having the epidural inserted especially since I could not see what was happening and had to sit still during the contractions. Eventually it was in and felt better almost immediately. Just the thought that it was in, made me feel better. Once the epidural was in, I was started on continuous foetal heart monitoring. I was exhausted so I slept for a couple of hours. Hearing my baby's heartbeat was reassuring. Another midwife introduced herself and stated that she would be supporting the first midwife. I now had two midwives, actually three, including myself. Every time they looked at the baby's heart trace I would also look to confirm their interpretation.

Labour continued for longer than expected, but Joshua was coping. The contractions slowed down so I was placed on an oxytocin drip to speed up labour. Joshua continued to cope. After 16 hours of labour the consultant obstetrician came in to introduce himself. He reviewed my progress and advised that a blood sample be taken from baby's scalp to check how he was coping. They took the blood sample but before the sample got tested it clotted and they could not use it. I was so upset. I felt helpless. They eventually took another sample and it showed that Joshua was coping and I was allowed to progress with labour. However, I was unhappy because I was unable to walk around as my legs were heavy and numb due to the epidural, and felt this was slowing things down.

The consultant obstetrician kept coming back every two hours to review my progress. It took about four hours to dilate between nine and 10 centimetres. When I was 20 hours into labour, the consultant came back to review me and stated that he would give me an hour before taking me to theatre for a Caesarean section. I was devastated. If I had a Caesarean section 20 hours ago I would be healing now, I thought to myself. I prayed so hard as having a Caesarean section would be the last straw for me. I begged Joshua to help me. We were so close. I am fully dilated so why isn't he coming out? I asked the midwives in despair. I kept looking at the heart trace for clues. Almost instantaneously Joshua moved. You could see my belly move as he moved. I felt like pushing I told the midwives. They checked and Joshua's birth was imminent. The midwives suggested that I rest for about thirty minutes before starting to push. I agreed, as I was exhausted. In time, I was ready to push and Joshua's head was crowning. His head was born but then I was asked to stop pushing. The cord was tight three times around his neck. If I continued pushing the cord could snap. The midwife had to clamp the cord and cut before he was fully out to enable him to be delivered. He was eventually born after 21 hours and 5 minutes of labour. I was excited that it was over. Looking back, I believe that Joshua's reduced movement in the last week of pregnancy was because he had inadvertently wound the cord round tightly around his neck so that he couldn't move freely.

> *'If you don't like something, change it. If you can't change it, change your attitude.'*
>
> Maya Angelou, Author and poet

Neonatal Intensive Care Unit

The midwives checked him out and eventually handed him to me. He looked all swollen, poor thing, like he'd just been in a boxing match. But two hours later he started grunting. The paediatrician came in to check him out and he was tired. He had respiratory distress, due to the long labour and his premature birth. Joshua was taken to the special care baby unit by the paediatrician and his dad accompanied him. I hate to say this but I was so happy when they took him to the neonatal unit as I was exhausted and felt he would be neglected if he stayed in my care overnight. I was transferred to the high dependency unit on the postnatal ward and slept like a baby overnight. I woke up very early the next morning and had a wash as I could now feel my legs. Then, with drip in hand, I was off to the special care baby unit. I was unprepared for what I saw. The night before, his dad had come back telling me that Joshua was stable. However, when I saw him he was ventilated – flat on his back looking so helpless. He had needles in his hands and a tube in his mouth. I began to wail. Despite previously working on a neonatal unit, it's different when it's your baby. The neonatologist (baby doctor) and nurses were very supportive and provided detailed explanation about his condition and the plan of care. Nonetheless, I didn't feel better.

Breast-feeding

The nurse caring for him provided me with his picture and advised me to go to the breast-feeding room and try to express some milk. Desperate to breastfeed as I was convinced it would give him the best start in life, I pumped and pumped. But nothing came. Joshua was kept on intravenous fluids all this time.

On the third day I felt feverish. My breasts felt like they would explode. You could see all the veins in them. It hurt like hell. The milk had come in. The textbooks simply cannot prepare you enough. Although it hurt, I was excited that I had milk. I pumped at first and then eventually put him to my breasts. Despite being a midwife and having the experience of supporting women to breastfeed, I felt like a total novice. However, Joshua was a natural. He suckled like he was experienced. But it hurt. No one adequately prepares you for the sensation you get with the letdown reflex (the automatic reflex that makes milk available in your breasts). After a nine-day stay in the neonatal unit, Joshua was discharged. I was elated. My difficult pregnancy and labour was over! If only. I spoke too soon.

> 'Things turn out best for the people who make the best of the way things turn out.'
>
> John Wooden, Former basketball player and coach

Not Another Setback – I Can't Handle This!

Joshua had been discharged, but I hadn't. My blood pressure was still high and my liver and kidney function was poor. The obstetricians were querying all sorts of medical conditions. I was terrified. I had scary thoughts that probably my role was just to bring Joshua to the world but not to raise him. I remember telling Joshua's dad that maybe I was dying. I had previously cared for women who had complications of pregnancy that resulted in organ failure and eventually death. Unsurprisingly this terrified him. He didn't say much but you could see it written all over his face. I kept having blood tests and other investigations.

Twelve days after Joshua was born, I felt contractions again. I initially thought that I could be expecting twins and I ran to the toilet and pulled the emergency cord. I heard a huge plop in the toilet. The midwife came in and there was blood everywhere. There was a massive clot that filled a litre jug. Instantly I felt physically better. It turned out I had retained some of the placenta and so my body acted as if I was still pregnant and the symptoms of pre-eclampsia continued. I had a scan later that day and my womb was clear. Over the next two days the symptoms disappeared and the blood test results improved. I was discharged from hospital when Joshua was 16 days old. Was I happy to see the back of hospital? I felt like a prisoner just let out after a long and hard sentence. Never had I imagined that I would enjoy inhaling the polluted air in London. But it was refreshing. I was free! But most importantly I was a mum of a beautiful baby boy – Joshua.

Sharing My Learning

Not all women will have the same experience of pregnancy, labour and childbirth as I have had. Everyone's experience will be different. However, it is important to be ready for the unexpected. Below are my tips for success:

- Change is a fact of life. We can't always predict change but we can prepare for it.
- Even when change is unplanned, embrace it. It will prove to be a learning experience.
- When things don't go according to plan, investigate why with a view to moving forward.
- Ask yourself: Can I control it? If not, then ask: Can I influence it? If the answer is still no then accept it!
- Always have a backup plan.
- You have control over your thoughts, so make them positive! It has benefits for you and your baby.
- When you find it difficult to think positively, ask yourself: What is good about my current situation?
- Eat a healthy, balanced diet.
- Exercise regularly.
- Have plenty of sleep and rest.
- Manage your expectations.
- Get informed.
- Advice is advice – you don't have to take it!
- Celebrate being pregnant.
- Remember – you can handle whatever situation you face!

Chapter 2

Who Are You?
Getting To Know Your Baby

Significant changes happen during pregnancies that create the foundations for babies' growth and development. In this chapter, I will introduce the key message of the book – to seek first to understand your baby, only then can you be understood. This has been adapted from one of Stephen Covey's *Seven Habits of Highly Effective People*, that has served me in developing and maintaining relationships. Becoming a parent is not just about you. To make parenting easier, try to step into your baby's shoes and see things through his eyes. Then you will understand the rationale for his behaviour and it will be easier to choose your response to it. I learned this the hard way as I kept putting my feelings before how my baby could be feeling. As I started to imagine how baby could be feeling in my womb I chose to do things that would help him feel better in my womb. This is not easy but with practice, it gets easier. You will also be better prepared to make healthy choices and provide empathic and responsive care for your baby.

Finding Out That You Are Pregnant

Finding out that you are pregnant can evoke a range of feelings in women. If the pregnancy is planned it can be an exciting experience. On the other hand, if it isn't then finding out that you are expecting a baby can be a negative experience as it was in my case. Whatever the case, it is important to process your feelings as they can impact on your baby. Step into your baby's shoes for a moment. Imagine you are the baby in your womb and that you can read your mum's feelings of dejection, regret and rejection. How would you feel? Unloved and unwanted! It is thus vital to regroup, come to some acceptance and move on with your pregnancy. This is not easy and as such, it is essential to have a good support network. Your partner, family and friends are often good sources of support at this time. So don't go it alone: use them! Rather than focusing on how the baby will limit your life, try to think of the ways a baby can enhance your life. Remember too, that many women would love to be in your shoes.

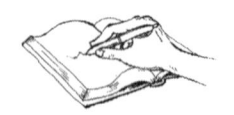

Please turn to the appendix and look for the heading *Finding Out That You are Expecting a Baby*.

Coming to Terms with Being Pregnant

Elisabeth Kübler-Ross developed a model called the Cycle of Grief that can be applied to people experiencing a life-altering event. It includes five stages and it is important to know these as they can help you in coming to terms with your pregnancy if it was not planned. You should note that these stages do not necessarily happen in sequence; neither do you spend equal times in each stage. Also, as everyone is unique in their responses to life events, you may not experience all of the five stages. But it may help you to understand your feelings, the way it did mine and also the rationale behind your reactions in order to enable you to deal with them.

The five stages are:

1. Shock and Denial

    When a person experiences a life-changing event, the first reaction is usually one of shock and complete disbelief. Then they move on to the denial phase. In the denial phase, the person refuses to accept the facts, information and reality, relating to the situation concerned. It's a defence mechanism and perfectly natural. This can be exhibited in different ways, for example not wanting to test for pregnancy even though you are experiencing signs of pregnancy, not wanting to have antenatal tests or checks, denying problems with pregnancy, etc. Remember that this is a normal reaction to an unplanned pregnancy. However, try not to get stuck in this phase as you and baby need care and attention.

2. Anger and Guilt

    There are several ways anger can show itself. People dealing with emotional upset can be angry with themselves, and/or with others, especially those close to them. They may also blame themselves. When a woman is expecting a baby, especially when it is unplanned, she may show anger towards her partner as she may feel that her life is on hold whilst her partner can continue with their life. Fear of the loss of independence may also cause a woman to become upset with her close relatives who are happy that she is expecting a baby. Again it is important not to get stuck in this phase and as such it is important to process your feelings to enable you to move on.

3. Bargaining

   A pregnant woman may begin to bargain or seek to negotiate a compromise. In my case, I did so when I decided to fast-track everything I was doing whilst I was pregnant without considering the effect it may have on the pregnancy. It was as if I was saying I would continue with my pregnancy, but only if I don't put other things in my life on hold. Although it appears that I had come to some form of acceptance, it was obvious that it was not sustainable due to the intense pressure it put me and my baby under, almost with disastrous consequences.

4. Depression and Despair

   This is also referred to as preparatory grief. It's like a dress rehearsal or trial run for the aftermath (Alan Chapman, 2006). However, this stage means different things to different people depending on who it involves. It is a sort of acceptance with emotional attachment. You begin to realise that you are indeed having a baby and almost start to mourn the loss of what motherhood may deny you. The feeling hits you hard and may leave you in a low mood for a period. Nonetheless, this is reassuring as it is natural to feel sadness, regret, fear, or uncertainty, as it shows that you have at least begun to accept the reality.

5. Acceptance

   In this stage, there is an emotional detachment and you become objective. You realise that baby is here to stay and the baby becomes the focus of your life. Almost nothing else matters. It is at this stage you start to tune in to your baby and prepare for life with a baby. Although it is important to reach this stage, remember

TUNE IN TO YOUR BABY

that the other stages are natural. Rushing through to acceptance without processing your feelings can cause a setback or relapse and may delay reaching some acceptance. It is also important to note that you may go through the cycle several times, especially if you have many setbacks in pregnancy as I did.

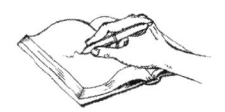

Please turn to the appendix and look for the heading *How Do I Feel about Being Pregnant? – Pregnancy Gains and Losses*

Once you come to terms with being pregnant, it is important to get good antenatal care. In order to access maternity care, inform your family doctor who will refer you to the midwife.

> *'If you would be loved, love, and be loveable.'*
> Benjamin Franklin, A founding father of the United States and polymath

First Trimester

Normal pregnancy lasts 40 weeks (nine months) and is divided into three trimesters. The first three months are often remembered for the unpleasant signs of pregnancy – nausea and/or vomiting (morning sickness), tender swollen breasts, tiredness and fatigue, altered sense of taste – food cravings or aversion, frequent urination, etc. However, it is a great time of activity and growth for the baby. By six to seven weeks, the baby's heart begins to beat. At about week nine the baby's eyes become more obvious and the first movements occur although the mum is unable to feel them. By 14 weeks after conception the baby is fully formed with all his organs, muscles, limbs and bones well developed. All that is required now is growth and maturity.

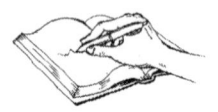

Please turn to the appendix and look for the heading *Calculating Baby's Due Date*

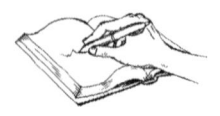

Please turn to the appendix and look for the heading – *Tune in to My Growth inside your Womb*

Booking Appointment

The midwife will offer an initial appointment which is called the booking appointment in the hospital, community clinic, doctor's surgery, or may visit you at home. This usually happens between 10 and 12 weeks but not before eight weeks as the risk of miscarriage is then still high. Be prepared to answer lots of questions, and complete several forms as the midwife needs to get a clear picture of your health, your partner's health and both of your families' medical history. At this appointment the midwife will use your last menstrual period to calculate baby's estimated date of delivery (E.D.D.). The midwife will ask about previous pregnancies and births as this will enable her to advise you about antenatal care and birth choices. You will be offered several tests to check you and

TUNE IN TO YOUR BABY

your baby's health. These will include blood and urine tests, screening tests and blood pressure checks. The midwife will also ask about your employment, lifestyle, where you would want to have your baby and birth choices. You will then be referred for a dating scan.

The First Scan (Dating Scan)

The first scan is often done by a sonographer (person carrying out the scan) between 10 and 14 weeks. It reveals a wealth of information that is vital for you and your baby's health and takes about twenty to thirty minutes. Measurements are taken that help date your pregnancy giving you a more accurate estimated date of delivery, check baby's gestation (baby's age in weeks), and can tell you how many babies you are expecting. The sonographer can see some of the baby's organs and would often point these out on the screen. You should be provided with a picture of the baby's image and a printed summary of the scan. Getting a picture of the baby and hearing a baby's heartbeat can help with bonding with the unborn baby as this confirms the realness of the baby.

For most women, the first scan is an exciting time – a time of celebration. However, this is not always the case as the scan can also reveal problems with the baby or loss of the baby. Therefore it is vital to have a support person with you when you attend this appointment.

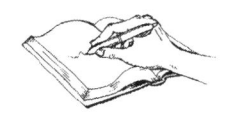

Please turn to the appendix and look for the heading – *My Baby's First Picture.*

The Second Trimester

The second trimester is often described as the 'honeymoon phase' as the unpleasant pregnancy signs often get better or disappear and the woman starts to enjoy being pregnant. As your pregnancy progresses, your baby might begin to seem more real. You might hear your baby's heartbeat at your antenatal appointments, and as your abdomen enlarges others may now know that you are pregnant. While you're adjusting to the changes in your body, this is also a time of rapid growth for the baby. Between 14 and 27 weeks the baby grows faster than at any other time in his life. It is at this time that the baby can distinguish between light and dark and starts to move more actively. Besides physical growth, baby also goes through rapid brain development.

Baby's Brain Development in the Womb

The development of a baby's brain in the womb is the foundation for life after birth. A baby's brain begins development three weeks after conception with the formation of the neural tube, which later forms the brain and spinal cord. By the 27th day, this tube is completely closed and its transformation into the brain and spinal cord has begun. The creation of neurons (brain or nerve cells) peaks before birth and some 100 billion are formed during the first five months of pregnancy. Just four weeks after conception, an unborn baby is already producing more than 8,000 new neurons every second, about half a million every minute (Dispenza, 2007).

Throughout the second trimester, the brain stem controls critical reflexes such as the baby's heartbeat, breathing, swallowing, sucking and blood pressure. By 27 weeks, the brain stem and its activities are for the most part mature. Your baby may hear your heart beating, your stomach rumbling or blood moving through the umbilical cord and may even be startled by loud noises. In the last three months of pregnancy, the brain stem and spinal cord grow steadily and are well-developed at birth.

Connect With Your Baby

For a baby's brain to grow to its full potential, it needs the right conditions – adequate nutrients, oxygen and a happy healthy place to live. Whilst in the womb, a baby responds to stimulus. When a baby is touched, talked to or hears a song, thousands of neurons (brain or nerve cells) are turned on and make connections with other brain cells and the connections get strengthened. As humans we need lots of connections that are well organised, just like traffic in a busy city – you get somewhere easier and faster if there are several ways to get there.

The environmental, physical and emotional being of the mother, all have a profound effect on foetal brain development and thus the behaviour of her baby. When the mum is stressed, the stress hormones affect the development of a baby's brain. Although babies can handle some stress, chronic stress affects the development of brain cells and hinders healthy connections between brain cells. By reducing the amount of stress she is under, a woman helps her baby. It is of utmost importance that a mum manages her thoughts and thinks happy, positive thoughts.

Also essential to a baby's brain development is the avoidance of poisonous substances. Cigarettes, alcohol and drug abuse can suppress growth of nerve cells leading to disabilities and brain impairments. Many infections can seriously threaten brain development such as German measles and chicken pox.

> *'Love is not only something you feel,
> it is something you do.'*
> David Wilkerson, Evangelist

Use It or Lose It!

A baby's developing brain creates many more brain cells than it will need. In the first three years of life, synapses (the gaps between brain cells) are created at an astonishing speed. By the time a child is 10, there are twice as many synapses as adults' brains with each neuron connected to as many as 15,000 brain cells. Whenever you repeat an activity with your baby, it increases the strength of the brain connections. The stronger connections will continue to be used by your baby over and over throughout life, and the weaker connections will eventually disappear. This is referred to as 'synaptic pruning' (Robinson, 2010). It begins at two years of age and is akin to how a gardener will prune plants in order to encourage health growth of the plant. You can liken this pruning process of nerve cells to a footpath. When it is well used it remains, but if it stops being used it eventually disappears. Hence the reason why they say use it or lose it! If the neurons are not used, they are pruned.

Twenty Week Scan

This scan is often referred to as the mid-pregnancy scan or anomaly scan as it takes a close look at your baby and your womb. It is often offered at between 18 and 21 weeks. The sonographer will check that your baby is developing well and talk you through the scan, highlighting the various organs; and look at where the placenta is lying in your womb. This is often an exciting time for the mum as your baby is much bigger and as such the scan is more detailed. You should also get a picture of your baby and a scan report. However, as the scan is to check that baby is growing normally, sometimes the scan can pick up problems with the baby. Thus, it is better to go with someone that can support you if any problems are detected.

You may also get to know the sex of your baby if you want to know and if your baby is lying in a position that enables the sonographer to determine baby's sex. Although you may not want to know your baby's sex, there are many benefits to finding this out. It can help you prepare for your baby's birth and life with your baby. Knowing the baby's sex can help with choosing colours for clothes, baby equipment and the nursery. It can also help with choosing your baby's name and connecting with baby.

What's In a Name?

A person's name is one of the easiest and most often used means of identifying him or her. Thus, deciding what to name your baby is one of the most important decisions you must make as an expectant parent. Knowing your baby's gender can help you and your partner (or any significant others) agree on your baby's name. Once you name your child, it is easier to connect with your baby even though he is still in your womb as you can then start to use the name and imagine him as a real person even before his birth. You and any significant others can call your baby by their name and bond intimately with him even before he is born.

I chose to give my baby a name as soon as I found out I was expecting a boy. I used his name from 21 weeks and it enabled me to develop a relationship with him. Being of African descent, naming a child is a significant event and a lot of thought goes into it. For an African, a name does not only represent a person's identity but is sometimes regarded as a promise, a blessing and/or a list of expectations. You can often tell the story surrounding a child's birth from his name. Once I gave my son his first name, I gave him an extra name every month I remained in hospital. Each name expressed the way I felt about remaining pregnant and my child being well. I used each name every time I spoke with him expressing how joyful I was for both of us being alive and well. I believed this strengthened my bond with him and to this day he enjoys hearing the story about his birth and the meaning of his names. However, I do realise that there are many customs and traditions surrounding childbirth and childrearing including superstitions about naming children before they are born. From my experience of caring for women in pregnancy and childbirth, some women also prefer not to know their baby's sex as they feel the surprise enables them to push their baby out in labour as they are eager to find out baby's sex. Thus, it is your choice as to whether to discover your baby's sex before birth and hence, deciding to name your child.

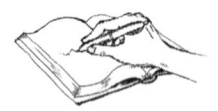

Please turn to the appendix and look for the heading *My Baby's Picture – At 20 weeks.*

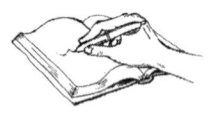

Please turn to the appendix and look for the heading *Naming My Baby.*

Communication – Look, Listen, and Feel

The key for a healthy and growing relationship is to keep the communication flowing. A relationship is a connection and exchange between people. Communication plays a vital role in exchanging ideas, wants, desires, feelings, and much more. Even though the baby cannot be seen, you can still establish communication with him. Imagine you were blind and you were speaking to a blind person, how would you communicate with them? You would have to rely on your other senses to communicate. Your unborn baby can listen and feel. You on the other hand can look, listen and feel. You can look at your baby's scan picture, your bump as it grows and how baby moves in your tummy. You can tell your baby how much you love him, what you dream for him, your intentions, fears and anxieties about birth and raising him. You can talk to your baby about anything and everything. Share your feelings with him because your baby feels them too. Remember that communicating is a two-way process. So be curious! Ask your baby questions about him, or ask the baby to do something you need them to do, such as staying inside of you or turning to a different position. Always allow time for a response. A long pause will do. As you feel him moving, smile and respond to him. Your smile will show in your tone of voice.

I recall on one occasion towards the end of my pregnancy, Joshua had a stretch and pushed one of his feet under my rib cage. It hurt so much and I tried to force his foot out but he stretched it even more. In despair, I pleaded with him to take his foot out because it was hurting me. I stroked my abdomen as I talked to him. To my relief, within a couple of minutes, although at the time it felt longer than that, he adjusted his position and took his foot out.

Pay attention to what your baby enjoys and doesn't enjoy. A baby usually becomes quiet in the womb when he is paying attention to something (Snelson, 2006). When babies are bothered by something, they will usually get extremely active as Joshua did whenever the midwife tried to feel my abdomen or listen to his heartbeat. However, remember that this is not a hard and fast rule. Before long your baby will get familiar with your voice and will try to interpret what you say by your tone. This will lead to you developing a relationship with your baby, which will continue after he is born.

Baby and Me Time

Thoughts become feelings. Feelings become actions. Actions become habits. Habits become routines. A neuron pathway is the channel through which information travels between the brain and body. The more times a neuron pathway is used, the easier and faster it will conduct an impulse along that same path. Each neuron has a central processing headquarter and a long sending fibre (or axon) over which it relays messages. Any thought or action repeated continuously builds little boutons (bumps) on the ends of the affected axons, making it easier to repeat the same thought or action. So if you find talking to your baby hard to do at first, you may want to get a small journal and begin to write in it regularly. Write in it as if you are having a conversation with your baby. Then read it out to him. By continuous repetition, this will eventually be a habit you will come to love and your baby will enjoy. Not only will this help you bond with your baby, but it will help preserve the memories and is a nice keepsake for your child when he is older. Select a convenient time to have some 'baby and me' time on a daily basis. By the time you have your baby this will be an established daily routine.

Regularly play music and notice the kind of music the baby likes. Read stories and rhymes to him and notice his response. After you eat a certain foods, monitor how your baby responds. It is worth noting that the way you feel emotionally, physically and mentally will have an impact on your baby's behaviour. Observe how your baby responds when you are happy, peaceful, upset or anxious. This will help you to understand the importance of reducing stress from your environment during pregnancy, during the birth and after baby is born.

Power of Touch

It is well recognised that a pat on the back or a peck on the cheek can make you feel special. However, there is growing evidence that touch, like massage, cuddles and hugs, can help premature babies gain weight, speed recovery from illness, and comfort us when we are afraid. The rationale behind it is that the skin is the body's largest organ, and when its receptors are stimulated, there is an increase in the release of oxytocin – the feel good hormone. At the same time there is a reduction in cortisol, the stress hormone.

You may have noticed that you frequently rub, pat or touch your bump throughout the day. Perhaps it is because as mothers to be, we unconsciously know that this is one way of physically reaching out and communicating with our unborn baby. You can make it a habit to touch your belly in different ways – stroking, patting, rubbing, etc. and try to converse with your baby when doing so. You can make tummy rubbing a frequent daily routine as you shower, or whilst moisturising your skin or whilst listening to music. If your baby responds, acknowledge it. Your baby will grow to love it.

> *'Blessed are the flexible, for they shall not be bent out of shape.'*
> Unknown

Baby's First Kick

Between 16 and 22 weeks the mum begins to feel baby moving and it is an exciting time. The initial sensations you'll notice aren't real kicks. Instead, some women describe the feeling as being like popcorn popping, bubbles blowing or butterflies in the stomach. If you don't feel any activity by 22 weeks, let your doctor or midwife know about it.

After a while, you'll begin to discern a pattern to your baby's movement and you'll know if something is not right. Make it a habit to sit and feel baby. Find a quiet time on a daily basis, sit still and count your baby's kicks. As he kicks, gently rub your abdomen and communicate with him. If he's not moving as often as he usually does, see your midwife urgently as your baby may be in distress.

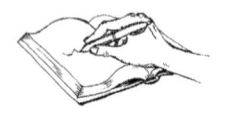

Please turn to the appendix and look for the heading *Baby and Me Time*.

The Last Trimester

The last three months is like the home straight, or last lap of pregnancy. Baby continues to grow in size as the organs mature which can pose problems for the expectant woman. The large size of the womb exerts pressure on other organs causing discomfort for the mum e.g. heartburn, frequent urination, shortness of breath, backache, swollen feet, tiredness, difficulty in sleeping. Despite these challenges, this phase of pregnancy is an exciting time for the expectant mum as she prepares for the birth of her baby and to become a parent.

Nesting

A woman may feel an intense desire to prepare a nest almost as a bird does in preparation for the arrival of her young. In this period, the expectant mum has a burst of energy and as she seeks to sort out her world and tie up loose ends before her baby is born. The act of nesting in pregnancy puts a woman in control and provides her with a sense of accomplishment prior to the birth of her infant. It is thought to be due to an increase in prolactin – the breast milk production hormone. I had my nesting experience at 29 weeks hence the reason for discussing it under the last trimester. However, it generally starts around the fifth month of pregnancy, although it can happen much earlier or later. Some women exhibit irrational compulsive behaviours such as painting the entire house, disinfecting the whole house, arranging cupboards in a particular way, etc. Do not be alarmed if your behaviour to prepare for your baby appears excessive. It just shows you care for your baby's arrival.

Prepare for Motherhood

Life with a baby is not easy, but giving some thought to what life with a baby may be like and some advance preparation will make the transition easier. Below are some suggestions you can try.

Imagine Life With a Baby – Prepare to Enjoy It!

Preparing for life with a baby prior to baby's birth can help you to cope with your new role as a mother. Prior to the birth of your baby try and visualise what life with a baby will look like. You can do this by positively pre-playing the outcome you desire. Doing this creates a strong command for your subconscious mind to help you achieve your goal. By focusing on what you want to achieve, your subconscious helps you to be the best you can be. It is your desire to be a good parent and enjoy the baby. As such, try to picture what you desire about parenting your new infant. Imagine what your day will be like, what you would enjoy about your new role and what may be challenging. Imagine that you will be a confident parent and meet your baby's needs such as feeding your baby.

Your Role as A Mother

Although motherhood is an exciting time, it is also a time when the realisation hits you that your life after having a baby would not be the same as your pre-baby life. The freedom and carefree days of your life before baby are behind. Now you have to be responsible for not only yourself but also a baby that is totally dependent on you. Even when you have planned to start a family, there will still be many challenging adjustments. Understanding and accepting the challenges of being a new parent can make the adjustment to parenthood easier and less stressful. Mourning the loss of your independent self is necessary for you to enjoy your new role. Therefore, avoid feeling guilty if you are feeling this way as it is a natural to feel this way.

Some You Lose, Some You Gain!

Although there are many things you will lose, there are also many things you will gain. So rather than focusing on your past, focus on your present. You can't go forward if you are looking back. You need to face the direction you are travelling in. You may find it useful to draw up a list of your losses and gains. As you do so try to imagine more benefits than drawbacks. Also try to think about ways that you will handle potential problems and who you will call on for support. Finally, remember that although you can prepare for your new role, you cannot prepare for every eventuality. Parenting is a role where you learn on the job!!

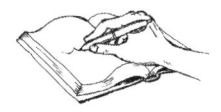

Please turn to the appendix and look for the heading *Prepare to Enjoy Motherhood.*

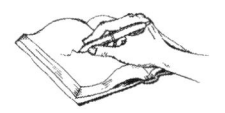

Please turn to the appendix and look for the heading *My Day Now and My Day after Baby is Here.*

Prepare to Breastfeed Whilst Pregnant

Breast-feeding has so many benefits for both mum and baby. It promotes bonding between a mum and her infant, is cheaper, convenient and also healthier for both mum and baby. Most importantly breast milk is designed for human babies and gives them a custom-made meal at each feed. Despite the numerous benefits, breast-feeding is not easy. Thus it is best to prepare for it prior to baby's birth. Below are some suggestions that you may want to try to prepare you for breast-feeding.

During pregnancy, try to attend a breast-feeding workshop or class. Your midwife can help you in finding local classes. Many women don't know how to breastfeed because they rarely see it done. So try to observe other mothers breast-feeding. You can do this by attending local breast-feeding cafés or groups and speak with other mothers that will be happy to answer your questions.

In my experience, I find that most mothers give up breast-feeding because they do not realise how hard and uncomfortable it will be in the initial phase. If you have not breast-fed a baby before, breast-feeding can feel strange at first until you get to grips with it. Often when you want to learn a skill, you will go to an expert to learn it. However, with breast-feeding, the baby who is a novice is learning to suckle from the mother, who is likewise a novice. It can feel like a case of blind leading the blind. But with support you both will soon be able to master the art of breast-feeding. Focusing on the benefits can help you succeed (I will discuss this further in the next chapter).

One key to successful breast-feeding is commitment. When you are committed to a cause you are unlikely to give up at the first hurdle. Despite initial problems you keep at it. This is why I believe successful breast-feeding is due to mindset. If you prepare yourself to succeed at it, you will. As the American industrialist Henry Ford once stated, 'If you think you can do a thing or think you can't do a thing, you're right.' It is important to think positively about your ability to breastfeed. Often I hear women say that they will get some formula just in case. If you already believe that you will fail before giving it a go, you are less likely to succeed.

In the last trimester of pregnancy, your baby laid down fat stores that he will break down for use after birth until breast-feeding is established. So there is no need to worry about your baby losing weight as long as your baby is healthy after birth and has no complications. So if you want to breastfeed, prepare your mind to enjoy it and you most likely will!

Preparing for Labour and Birth

The due date is fast approaching and with each passing day you are preparing for the arrival of your baby. Below is a list of things that you may want to consider in getting ready for labour and baby's birth. The topics are not exhaustive but will focus on you and your baby and empower you to make the right choices for both of you.

Antenatal Classes

Antenatal classes aim to get you ready for labour, birth, and early parenthood. They help you focus on your pregnancy and prepare for labour and birth. They are also a great place to meet other parents-to-be who may form part of your support network during pregnancy and after baby is born.

Topics covered in antenatal classes usually include signs of labour, when to call the midwife or go into hospital, pain relief, what happens in labour, birth positions, breathing and relaxation techniques, complications of labour and childbirth and how these are managed, breast-feeding, and preparation for life with a baby.

Although these classes are not compulsory, it is recommended that you attend them as it better prepares you for labour and delivery. Attending these classes with your birthing partner will enable you and your partner to get informed and clarify any misconceptions you might have about your labour and baby's birth. It is also advisable to attend a tour of the unit you will be having your baby at to familiarise yourself with its atmosphere. Ask your midwife about local antenatal classes.

Birth Planning

A *birth plan* is a way for you to communicate your wishes to the midwives and doctors that will care for you in labour. It informs them about your wishes for labour and delivery of your baby. In it you can outline your preferences and what you want to avoid.

Writing a birth plan also empowers you and gives you some control over decisions that need to be made. It ensures that the midwife and your birthing partner are aware of your preferences for the birth of your baby.

The following is a list of things you may want to include in Your Birth Plan.

Birthing Partner	• Who will be your birthing partner? • When do you want them with you? • Have you shared your Birth Plan with them?
First Stage of Labour:	
Choice of professional	• Do you prefer to be only cared for by women? • Do you mind if students are present?
Monitoring baby's heart	• How often do you want baby's heart to be monitored if everything is alright with baby: intermittently or continuously?
Mobility	• How mobile do you want to be in labour?
Labour position	• Would you want to use any special birthing equipment such as mats, beanbags, balls, birthing chair, etc.?
Birth pool	• Use of bath/ shower/pool: do you want to use it for labour only or would you want to give birth in it?
Pain relief	• What do you want for pain relief? List the order of pain relief methods. • What methods of pain relief do you want to avoid?
Speeding up labour	• Would you want interventions to speed up labour such as breaking your waters?

Second Stage of Labour: (Whilst baby is being delivered)	
Birth position	• Do you want to remain upright? On all fours? Lying in bed?
Episiotomy	• How do you feel about having an episiotomy?
Delivery of the baby	• Do you want baby delivered on to your tummy or do want baby to be cleaned first?
	• Would you want your partner to be actively involved in the delivery of the baby?
Assisted Delivery	• Do you have a preference for forceps or vacuum delivery?
Third Stage of Labour: (Delivery of the Placenta)	
Management	• Do you want a natural or managed delivery of the placenta?
	• Do you want your partner to cut the cord?
After the Birth:	
Vitamin K	• Do you want baby to have it?
	• If so, orally or by injection?
Feeding baby	• How do you plan to feed your baby?
Other things	• Do you need a special diet?
	• Are there any special religious customs you wish to be observed?

The above list is not exhaustive. If there are any issues not covered that you feel strongly about, then discuss them with your midwife.

If you need assistance with writing a birth plan, talk to your midwife who can assist you with writing one. And when you've written your birth plan, remember to include it in your hand held notes or take it with you to hospital or the Birth Centre.

Remember that it is just a plan and it needs to be flexible. You need to acknowledge that things may not go as planned due to complications of labour and delivery. So I always suggest that my clients have a backup plan – a Plan A, Plan B, Plan C – or more, as many as you feel you need. I find it helps you to manage disappointment and cope with setbacks especially if things don't go exactly as planned. It definitely helped me!

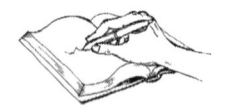

Please turn to the appendix and look for the heading *Planning My Baby's Birth*.

> 'A very small degree of hope is sufficient to cause the birth of love.'
> Stendhal, Writer

Labour

Pain Relief

Until you go into labour, you will not know how it will feel for you. Even if you have had a baby before, every pregnancy and birth is unique. One thing is sure – it will hurt! That is why it is called labour. Pain thresholds differ from person to person and as such some women may cope with little or no pain relief, whilst others may want labour to be almost pain-free. Below is a list of the different kinds of pain relief. Please discuss these options with your midwife as this book will not cover these.

Medical Pain Relief
- Epidural
- Mobile epidural
- Spinals
- Pethidine
- Meptid
- Entonox (gas and air)
- TENS – Transcutaneous Electronic Nerve Stimulation

Natural Methods of Pain Relief
- Breathing and relaxation
- Water
- Warmth
- Massage
- Active birth positions

In this book I will focus mainly on how your mindset can help you to cope with labour. I discovered this from my experience of working as a community midwife assisting pregnant women with delivering their babies at home. I learned that preparing your mind for labour can help you cope with the pain of a normal delivery. This was further affirmed by the way I coped with my personal experience of labour.

> *'If you fail to plan you are planning to fail.'*
> Benjamin Franklin, A founding father of the United States and polymath

Mindset

Before I went into labour I had observed and cared for several women in labour. So I knew labour would be hard work. Some women quietly coped with the pain, whilst others screamed intensely. So I guessed the pain would be intense and imagined that I would be undergoing the worst pain ever. I had had a couple of operations in the past and I expected the pain to be worse than that. In the pre-labour phase, I mobilised or walked all over the labour ward. For me this was freedom as I had been bed-bound for so many months. If you had asked me then to run the marathon, I believe I could. At the time, anything was better than lying in a hospital bed. In my head I had prepared to endure a number of hours of pain. My labour progressed very well in the earlier stages so that at 3cm dilated I thought my labour would last another eight hours (an hour for each centimetre of the cervix dilating and an hour for pushing baby out). When my baby was not born in eight hours, I was so downhearted that I gave up! The pain did not intensify, but I just felt I could not progress with labour without additional pain relief. Looking back, I believe that if I had prepared myself for a 20-hour labour, I would have handled it without extra pain relief.

The rationale for this is because of the relationship between thoughts and feelings – *you feel the way you think!* This is one of the core concepts of Cognitive Behavioural Therapy (CBT) – a form of therapy that aims to help change the way that a person thinks, feels and behaves. In view of this, it is important to manage your thoughts. Preparing your mind that labour will be long and may be very painful will help you manage your feelings.

One's outlook also has a bearing. I will demonstrate this by using the glass half empty or glass half full analogy. Instead of thinking that each contraction was one contraction less to the birth of my baby, I thought, not another one! Exactly the same contraction, but different interpretations! Striving to focus on the positive aspect of the pain such as it being productive in nature, may help you to cope with it.

You probably have heard the phrase 'what you see is what you get'. Our minds have an amazing ability and play an important role in the creation of our experiences. *Visualisation* is a key to creating your birth experience, as it can harness the power of your subconscious mind to achieve your dream of having a successful delivery. By using your brain's ability to visualise – 'seeing' what your body *should* be doing, you can direct your body and programme your mind in a certain way to gain positive results such as coping with the pain of labour to enable the birth of your baby. Visualising yourself having a normal delivery and then holding your baby can help you through the pain of childbirth.

Relaxation is also vital. The more you relax in labour, the less tense you will become. Your body will work better giving you more energy for your baby's birth. Your muscles tense in response to stress and anxiety. When tension is prolonged, you get tired and energy is wasted. If you are stressed or anxious in labour, your body produces fight-or-flight hormones, such as adrenaline which reduce the flow of blood to your womb. Your womb needs a good blood flow to help it contract strongly. Preventing stress in labour encourages your body to produce more oxytocin - a hormone that helps with labour and acts as a natural pain killer.

Finally, I want to highlight the baby's role in the birth process. Having supported women in the delivery of their stillborn babies, I have come to realise the role a baby has to play in being delivered. A baby plays an active role in its birth and works with his mum's contractions to manoeuvre his journey through the birth canal. If you have formed a relationship with your unborn baby you can communicate with him alerting him that it is time to come out and urging him to work with you through the pain. I did this and I believe that it worked for me. However, I am not suggesting that it will work for you, but to give it a try as you will only know if it does if you try it.

What if Things Don't go According to Plan?

Having made a birth plan, an expectant mum hopes the birth of her baby goes to plan. However, this is not always the case. I will briefly discuss some of these, but more importantly I will suggest some ways that you can cope if you find yourself in any of these situations.

Prematurity

Going into labour before the baby's due date can lead to the premature birth of your baby but does not always have to. Sometimes drugs can be given to stop early contractions or a stitch may be inserted into the cervix (the neck of the womb) to keep it closed. Causes of premature labour include weakness of the cervix, the waters breaking before the due date, vaginal bleeding and contracting before the baby is due to be born. In some cases, doctors may start labour early because the baby is not growing well in the womb.

Your baby is premature if he arrives before you are 37 weeks pregnant. About 8 per cent of babies are born prematurely with most premature babies arriving after 28 weeks of pregnancy (Tommy's) and having a good chance of surviving and growing up healthy. Notwithstanding this, going into labour early can be stressful for a pregnant woman due to its suddenness and the unpreparedness of the expectant mother. This can be made worse by unfamiliarity with the hospital environment, lack of control of the mum over the situation and the need to make quick decisions about her health and that of her unborn baby. In their efforts to stop the labour and early birth of baby, health care professionals may provide information that requires a quick response from the mum, but they may not be able to provide her with adequate support. It is therefore useful for her to consider her options, and what she would do, before she goes into premature labour.

Induction of Labour

Although it is better for labour to start naturally, it can be started artificially if the baby has gone past his due date, if the waters have broken but there are no contractions, or if there is any risk to the mum's or baby's health, for example if the mum has high blood pressure or if the baby is not growing well in the womb. The induction of labour is always planned in advance so you should be given a detailed explanation about what the process should involve and be given the opportunity to ask questions. Once labour is started, it often progresses normally. However, induced labour is usually more painful than normal labour, so it is useful to discuss your pain relief options in advance and prepare yourself mentally to cope with it

Instrumental Delivery – Forceps Delivery or Vacuum Extraction

As the name implies, sometimes babies may need assistance during birth. Perhaps because they have got into an awkward position, or are getting distressed with labour, or the contractions are not strong enough, or the mum is too tired to push baby out. Instruments are used to assist the delivery of the baby – forceps or vacuum extraction. Sometimes a cut is made to the skin of the perineum (the area between your vagina and back passage) to make the opening bigger. This is called an episiotomy. Forceps are placed around the baby's head to assist the baby's birth. With vacuum delivery, a suction cap is placed on the baby's head to help him out.

Although assisted deliveries cannot always be prevented, there are a few things that you can do that may reduce the need for you to have one, such as adopting upright positions in labour, not having an epidural so that you are able to mobilise, and having a continuous support person in labour to help you cope with the pain. In the eventuality that you do have to have an assisted delivery ensure that you understand what the procedure involves.

Caesarean Section

Despite planning to have a normal delivery, sometimes a Caesarean section is the safest way to deliver the baby as speedy delivery is required in order not to compromise your health or that of your baby. This involves cutting through the abdomen and the womb to get your baby out. Caesarean sections may be planned if the doctors deem it too dangerous for you or the baby to go into labour. An emergency Caesarean section may be required if complications develop in labour and baby's delivery needs to be expedited. If you require a planned Caesarean section ensure that you are given ample opportunity to ask questions as this will enable you to have more control over decision making. Notwithstanding this, if you require an emergency Caesarean section, ensure that you ask why it is needed and if there are any possible side effects.

Many women express disappointment when they plan to have a normal delivery and they do not. However, not having a normal delivery is not a failure on your part. If you feel this way, it is important to talk about how you feel as it will help you deal with it and process your feelings. It is important to realise that you are not alone. Many women often feel like this when the outcome of pregnancy is different from what they expected. It is often said that it's good to talk, so talk with the obstetrician, midwives and your health visitor. Debrief with them and go over what happened. It helps with the healing process and gives closure to the events surrounding the pregnancy and birth of your baby. Remember too, that just because you did not have a normal delivery on this occasion does not mean that you won't if you decide to have another baby.

Although we plan for a normal pregnancy, labour and delivery this does not guarantee that we will have one. Pregnancy, labour and birth are all unpredictable. The goal of all three is that you have a healthy mum and baby at the end of it. So if you and your baby are healthy, you have succeeded. This is one time I strongly believe that it is the destination that matters and not the journey. If you learned from the journey, it's a bonus! My pregnancy and birth journey were very tough, but my destination – my baby's health and mine – was what mattered most. Celebrate your achievement – you are a mum now!

Problems After the Birth of Your Baby

Sometimes things go to plan in labour and delivery but go wrong after the birth of the baby. This can either be with you or the baby.

Sick Child

You have finally had your baby and although you may be exhausted, you are overjoyed – the birth is over and you are a proud mother. Sometimes this feeling does not last as your baby is whisked away, separated from you at birth and may require a stay in the special care baby unit. This may be very a difficult and nerve-wracking experience, especially if you are not able to be with your baby. Ask your partner or support person to accompany your baby and if possible take a picture of him. You can also ask that the special care baby unit staff provide you with a picture for you to bond with your baby. As soon as you can, try to see your baby. It may be hard at first especially if your baby requires intensive care. If your baby is in an incubator or on machines, ask the unit staff to explain what each machine is for. Try to get involved in your baby's care and ask for help in handling your baby. Keep communicating with your baby. Your baby will recognise your voice if you have been regularly talking with him in pregnancy. Touch him, stroke him and continue to tell him how much you love him. Encourage him to get better and let him know how much you are looking forward to his recovery. As he continues to progress let him know how he is progressing. As soon as you are able to, start skin-to-skin contact. Lying on your chest will remind him of your heartbeat which he became accustomed to in your womb. Breast-feeding is especially important for premature babies. So if you plan to breastfeed, get the unit staff to assist you with expressing breast milk. Having a picture of your baby with you and thinking positive thoughts about your baby when you are expressing can help with the flow of milk.

Ensure you speak with the neonatologist about your baby's progress and plan of care. Ask as many questions as you need to ensure you understand what is happening to your baby. Express your wishes to the neonatologist so that you are involved in the plan of care. Also make sure that you get support from your partner, family and relevant others as this can be a difficult time for you. Other parents with babies in the Special Care Baby Unit can also provide invaluable support and can be added to your support network when baby is well enough to go home.

Look after yourself by getting adequate sleep, eating well and keeping hydrated. Remember to take each day as it comes and manage your thoughts by thinking positively.

TUNE IN TO YOUR BABY

> *'Begin at once to imagine it the way you want it to be – and move into that. Check every thought, word and action that does not fall into harmony with that. Move away from those.'*
>
> Neale Donald Walsch, Author

Sick Mum

Sometimes, the baby is well but you are not. I spent a few hours after the birth of my baby in the high dependency unit as my blood pressure was still elevated. This was so difficult because I was separated from my baby who was in the special care baby unit. I wondered what was happening to him as I knew he was not well. Despite not wanting to be separated from my son, I had to try to focus on the benefits of my situation. I was not well and that was the reason I needed special attention. I had a picture of my baby that his dad had taken with his phone so I thought about him and felt I had to get well for him.

Two weeks later, I was still unwell. During this period, it was very difficult to manage my thoughts. Even though I eventually got to see my baby regularly I was terribly scared that I may die as no one knew why I remained unwell. The support of my loved ones was very important at this time. I had to take every passing day as it came. Even though I was unwell I visualised getting better and going home with my baby and this I believed pulled me through.

It can be very difficult to bond with your baby after birth, if you are unwell. You may feel disappointed that you are not able to provide care for your baby. However, be kind to yourself. Ensure the health care professionals give you adequate information about your condition, the plan of care and the prognosis (the predicted outcome). Get involved in your care as much as possible. Try to trust those who are caring for your baby. Manage your thoughts and endeavour to *think* positively so that you can *feel* positive. Eventually you will be able to be reunited with your baby and show him how much you love him.

Sharing My Learning

- Try to *step into your baby's shoes* and see things through his eyes. Then you will understand the rationale for his behaviour and it will be easier to choose your response to it.
- If you are having difficulty coming to terms with your pregnancy, rather than focusing on how the baby will limit your life, try to think of the ways he can enhance it.
- Ensure you get antenatal care.
- Track your baby's growth and development in your womb.
- Try to get a picture of the baby at the scan appointment and listen to the baby's heartbeat at antenatal appointments as it can help with bonding with your unborn baby.
- Once you know your baby's sex, name your baby and use his name in your daily conversations.
- Make it a habit to communicate regularly with your unborn baby. Incorporate 'baby and me' time into your daily routine.
- Communicate with baby by *looking* (observing baby's movements), *listening* (allowing baby to respond) and *feeling* (rubbing your abdomen).
- Play music and say rhymes to your baby. Share your dreams and your fears. Imagine how it is for baby in the womb – be curious about your baby!
- Let baby know how it will be outside the womb. Prepare baby for life outside the womb. Let baby know how you are preparing for his birth.
- Let baby know why you love him.

- Plan your birth but remember that it is just a plan: be flexible!
- Prepare your mind for labour and childbirth.
- Remember that not having a normal delivery is not failure on your part!
- If there are any complications, ask your health care providers to inform you about you and/or your baby's care and involve you in it.
- If things don't go as planned, remember to debrief with your health care professionals.
- Ensure you have support through pregnancy, labour, childbirth and after baby is born.
- Towards the end of your pregnancy, imagine life with a new baby: what's going to be challenging? What's going to be great about it? Prepare to enjoy life with your baby.
- Remember that whatever happens in pregnancy, labour, childbirth and after baby is born, you can handle it!

Chapter 3
I've Had My Baby What Do I Do Next?

You've had your baby and probably feel special, excited and proud of your new role. Sometimes this feeling does not last for long especially as this new role brings with it a huge responsibility. The excitement of having a baby can be overwhelming and then you get discharged home and all of a sudden you feel all alone as it dawns on you that your newborn baby is totally dependent on you. You want to do the best for your baby, but you are unsure what to do, which causes you some anxiety. You are surrounded by people all claiming to be experts – professionals, mothers, sisters, other family members and friends, but their advice leaves you confused because it is conflicting. How will you determine what to do?

It is important to emphasise that you are not alone! Despite being a nurse and midwife, I felt that way. After spending such a long time as a patient in hospital, although I was ecstatic to be discharged from hospital I felt very anxious about the next steps regarding caring for my baby. I had experienced such a difficult pregnancy, labour and birth, that I wanted to make up for it after Joshua's birth. I had received a lot of support from the hospital staff, but I felt unsure if I would be able to meet his needs by myself. Because Joshua was also premature I was worried that I may accidentally harm him as he was so small and looked very fragile. I wanted the best for him but doubted my ability to provide for his needs.

It is vital to stress that the feelings of anxiety that you experience as a new mum are very natural but more importantly, it shows that you care! Once again, I believe the baby can help you answer what to do next. To do this however, you will have to step into your baby's shoes and try to see things through his eyes. Your baby cannot talk and this can make it difficult for you to find out what his needs are. However, a baby communicates in other ways without using speech. Getting his perspective can also enable you to determine what your baby needs.

Let's start by sharing your baby's experience of labour and delivery.

> 'The ability to discipline yourself to delay gratification in the short term in order to enjoy greater rewards in the long term is the indispensable prerequisite for success.'
>
> Brian Tracy, Author and motivational speaker

Labour and Birth Through Your Baby's Eyes

Labour starts for you and it is painful. But how does it feel for your baby? Let's step inside your womb and try to relive your baby's journey to the world through the birth canal. This could be a long while especially if you have a long labour. The first stage of labour usually lasts about 12–14 hours, but can last much longer, especially in a woman expecting her first baby. Close your eyes and try to use your imagination. Let it run free. All you know is inside the womb. You've never seen the outside world. You are upside down. All enclosed in your mum's womb. The peaceful atmosphere has been interrupted. All of a sudden there is a tight sensation, you feel squeezed (contraction). You've felt this before. Your mum had Braxton Hicks contractions (contractions that sometimes start in pregnancy but don't cause discomfort). But this tightening and squeezing is nothing like you've experienced before. After about 30–40 seconds the tightening and squeezing stops. Wow, you're glad it's over. Another 10 minutes or so pass, and then you feel it again! Then another one, in another 10 minutes. Just as you start to get used to the tightening and squeezing, they become more intense, come more often and they last so much longer. They are now lasting for 60-90 seconds and coming every 3–4 minutes. Your mum's heart rate is racing. Every so often you feel a prod (foetal heart rate monitor transducer) and no matter how much you try to move away, it keeps following you. Soon after you feel the prod, you start to hear steady beating (the baby's heart beat through the foetal heart monitor) from the outside. After a few hours the water breaks. Your mum does not appear comfortable. She sounds distressed. She is breathing heavily. What's going to happen next, you wonder. Every so often you feel a couple of fingers around your head or running along your scalp (internal examinations). Hours pass, and as labour continues, the tightening and squeezing push you down your mum's pelvis. Eventually the cervix is fully dilated and your head hits your mum's pelvic floor. The tightening and contractions are much stronger, more frequent and lasting longer. Your mum starts to bear down, using her diaphragm and abdominal muscles to push you down the birth canal. You've got no choice, you've got to come out of the womb, but that's all you know. You're distressed! Life as you know it has changed. Eventually after several hours (if your mum is delivering her first baby) of you being squeezed by your mum's contractions and bearing down, you are born into a strange environment. You can't see clearly. But the lights are bright and you don't recognise anyone. The cord connecting you to your mum is cut off and clamped. You are wet and so you are dried off, quickly checked by another strange person and are handed to your mum in a rough towel for you to be cuddled by her. You feel so disoriented and eventually cry. The events of the last few hours have left you in a state of shock so you have a glazed look or are so exhausted that you go off to sleep.

And that's a normal delivery! When things don't go to plan, for instance if labour progresses for longer than planned, or you don't go into labour naturally, some interventions are performed. Sometimes labour is induced or sped up with drugs such as artificial oxytocin which can bring on stronger contractions, hence stronger tightening and squeezing is felt by the baby as the womb contracts. According to Melton (2010), the use of artificial oxytocin can feel like an unrelenting assault with no pauses for the baby. This is because artificial oxytocin can eliminate the natural spaces between contractions, causing exhaustion, stress and trauma, resulting in a baby and then child who has a very revved nervous system and can't stop or relax. Other interventions include continuous foetal heart rate monitoring from the mum's abdomen, the use of a probe attached to the baby's scalp to hear baby's heart rate, or a blood sample taken from the baby's head. Imagine what the baby feels, especially as they don't know what is happening or why.

Then if you require an assisted delivery, the baby either has a suction cap attached to the crown of his head or forceps around his head and is gently pulled out by the doctor as mum pushes with the contractions.

If it's a Caesarean section, the womb is cut open and baby is quickly pulled out of it and the obstetrician hands baby over to the paediatrician (doctor that cares for children) who checks baby out thoroughly before handing baby to mum or mum's birthing partner. Often in an emergency Caesarean section the baby will need to be pulled out of the birth canal backwards, as baby has already travelled down it. How they are lifted out, pushed or pulled can form part of a baby's birth imprint (Melton, 2010). After the baby is delivered, there is an immediate need to quickly clear out his lungs. In a normal birth the physical action of going through the birth canal squeezes the fluids out of his lungs so that he can take his first breath when he is born. With a Caesarean section, a baby's lungs are still full of fluids so the secretions have to be sucked out. This often means putting a tube down their throat, which can be quite traumatic for him. The baby is also born into noisy surroundings with bright lights in the presence of strange people and sounds. No wonder baby looks so shell-shocked after birth. It's been a traumatic experience for mum, but even more so for baby as he does not understand what is happening and why.

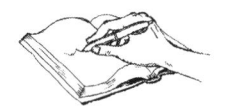

Please turn to the appendix and look for the heading *Feel Your Baby's Journey to the World*.

What a Hard Life!

For a baby, life outside the womb is hard. Inside his mum's womb everything was done almost automatically. Your baby never felt signs of hunger as he did not need to use his gastrointestinal tract (gut). Your baby relied solely on you for nutrition. He got nourished through the placenta which was rich in blood supply. Blood containing nutrients and oxygen were taken to the placenta, and then from the placenta to the baby via the umbilical cord. Your baby was nourished and waste products were carried out of the baby through the cord back to the placenta where your blood picked them up and carried them away. Your unborn baby's lungs were also not used in the womb – he received oxygen via the placenta. Towards the end of pregnancy, your unborn baby started to practise breathing movements. When your baby was born and the cord was cut, a rapid change in your baby's body began. His lungs filled with air and started to work, and he became able to eat with his mouth, digest food and get rid of wastes through his back passage. What a change for your baby: nutrition and oxygenation which were once effortless for him have now become much harder.

Also, in the womb, your baby was in his little secure container. He was warm, cosy, he always heard your heartbeat and was reassured by it. He didn't have to cry – well he couldn't. He just had to move if he was uncomfortable and you probably stroked him, talked to him and showed you cared about him. Now this cushy life has ended and he'll have to work harder for everything he needs for his survival. No wonder he cries. He protests, I'm not used to this life and I don't like it! Try to put yourself in your baby's shoes. Be empathic and try to feel for your baby! You probably would act the same way if you found yourself in similar conditions.

Replicate the Womb Conditions for Baby Outside the Womb

Your baby would love to go back inside your womb. However, that cannot happen. So as a mother, try the next best thing by creating the same conditions that your baby is used to outside the womb. In your womb it was not too bright so use dim lights until your baby adjusts to brighter lights. In your womb it was cosy, so try to give baby lots of hugs and cuddles. Skin-to-skin contact can also help. Early skin-to-skin contact begins immediately after birth by placing the naked newborn baby prone on the mum's bare chest. This intimate contact within the first hours of life may facilitate maternal-infant behaviour and interactions through sensory stimuli such as touch, warmth, and odour. It is also a critical component for successful breast-feeding initiation. Several studies have highlighted the benefits of skin-to-skin contact for the baby. He is more likely to latch on to the breast well, more likely to breastfeed exclusively for longer, less likely to cry, more able to regulate his body temperature, maintain his heart rate, respiratory rate and blood pressure and maintains higher blood sugar. Immediately after birth, skin-to-skin contact also allows the baby to get used to the mum's bacteria (Newman, 2009).

Skin-to-skin contact is especially beneficial for premature infants and is often called kangaroo care. The name is derived from how marsupials, like a kangaroo, carry their young in their pouch. This form of care was initially developed to care for premature infants where incubators were not available. As a premature baby should still be in his mum's womb, kangaroo care seeks to provide restored closeness of the newborn with his mum by placing the infant in direct skin to skin contact with her. Because Joshua was premature, I used this method of care, which kept him warm and safe. Even after discharge, I continued to use skin to skin. I would also regularly carry him in a sling in front of me. When he was about a month old, being an African, I started to put him on my back and tie him to my back with a long piece of cloth. I remember the first time I put him on my back. I was so scared that I would drop him that I sat on the bed just in case. Before long, I became an expert at this and he would assist me to put him on my back. He felt so warm and secure, as he could hear my heart beat and shortly after I put him on my back he would sleep. Very rarely did he cry when he was on my back. I believe that this contributed to his easy transition to life outside the womb. However, I am in no way saying that you have to put your baby on your back as there is no clinical evidence to support this practice. Skin-to-skin or close contact is what matters for your baby.

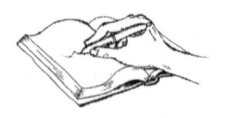

Please turn to the appendix and look for the heading *Mimic the Womb, Outside the Womb*.

Use Your Baby's Senses

It's difficult for a mum to know exactly what her newborn is feeling. However, if you pay close attention to your baby's responses to light, noise, and touch, you can decipher how your baby's senses are developing.

Your newborn infant can see about a distance of about 20 to 30cm, and focus when looking up from your arms. Although your newborn can see distant objects, they cannot focus on them. It takes about six months for the newborn to see across a room. Notwithstanding this, newborn babies are very sensitive to bright light; as such maintain dim lights to encourage your baby to open his eyes. Newborn babies love human faces. So make time to stare at your baby whilst he stares back at you. I remember doing this for long periods when Joshua was a few weeks old. As his vision got clearer, you could almost imagine his thoughts as he first clearly saw my face. His facial expression said it all. Without speech, I could hear him think, so that's what you look like! It was a lovely feeling.

Babies smile from birth. But in the early weeks, this is usually an automatic behaviour. By about 4–6 weeks, your baby will be able to give you a responsive smile (a smile back when you smile at him). When this happens, smile back, thank and praise him for it so that he will know that you are pleased with his behaviour. After human faces, newborn babies like to look at bright colours, contrasting patterns, and movement. They find black-and-white pictures or toys more attractive than objects or pictures with lots of similar colours. When quiet and alert, your baby should be able to follow the slow movement of your face or an interesting object. Therefore, in order to prevent your baby from getting bored, introduce him to new objects but don't overstimulate him as he may get overwhelmed.

By the time he is born, a baby's hearing is fully developed. If you have established a relationship with your baby in pregnancy, he will recognise your voice and its tone. If you have made it a habit to regularly communicate with your baby, your baby will feel secure as you explain to him why he had to come out of your womb. When you talk to your baby, ensure that it is quiet, so that your baby can have your full attention without distraction from background noise. Assure your baby that you can imagine how it feels for him – how traumatised labour must have made him feel; how you know he must want to go back to life inside your womb, but he can't. Let him know that you will endeavour to help him settle into life outside the womb and how much you love him. Introduce him to the other members of his family – father, siblings, grandparents, and any other relevant others. He may recognise their voices too.

Touch is powerful, and is extremely important for your baby, as it is for most humans. Through touch, babies learn a lot about their surroundings. So stroke him whilst talking to him. Having come from a warm environment before birth, cuddles will help keep him warm. Cuddles will also ensure that your baby hears your heart beating. He'll recognise it. It will remind him of when he was in your womb and make him feel safe. With almost every touch a newborn is learning about life, so provide lots of tender kisses and your little one will soon find the world a comforting place to be. Baby massage can be useful too, for you and baby. The gentle rhythmic stroking helps in the release of oxytocin and helps baby relax and sleep better.

> *'There are no secrets to success. It is the result of preparation, hard work, and learning from failure.'*
>
> Colin Powell, American Statesman

Reading and Responding to Your Baby's Cues

You may have lots of questions about how you are caring for your baby and worry about whether what you are doing is right for your baby. But don't worry – you are not alone. Many parents feel the same. They are concerned that they may not be able to ascertain their baby's needs because their little one cannot speak. How then can you know what your baby needs are? In order to understand your baby, it is essential to learn how your baby lets you know what he needs and how he is feeling. However, it is also important to remember that every baby is unique. As such getting it 'right' for your baby will be different from other babies. Your baby will have his own way of letting you know how best to care for him.

From birth, babies have certain behaviours that help them to communicate with you and be sociable. As your baby can't speak, your baby will communicate with you mainly using body language. These are called cues. It is vital to ensure that you take time to observe baby and look at what he does in order to read these cues. When you read your baby's cues and respond quickly to his needs, your baby will feel secure and the bond between you and him will be strengthened.

Your baby will employ approach cues when he wants to interact with you. He will look at you, reach towards you, smile at you, babble and talk to you and his eyes are usually bright and wide. This is often a good time to talk to, play with and feed your baby (UI Maternity Centre, 2004).

When your baby is tired, needs a break from you or is distressed, he will use withdrawal cues. He will often turn or pull away, arch his back, whine or fuss, squirm or kick, cry or sometimes vomit. He may need to stop eating, playing, or being held. Sometimes your baby may get bored by a certain activity and require a change from what is happening. He may do this by looking away, turning his head away, yawning, having a dull-looking expression or putting his hands up to his face. Often when baby needs a change of pace, he becomes restless or more active (Chitty, et al, 2007).

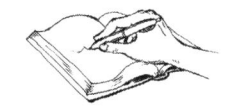

Please turn to the appendix and look for the heading *Your Baby's Cues.*

Reading and Responding to Your Baby's States

During the course of each day your baby will move through different levels of sleepiness and wakefulness. These are called 'states'. By learning to tell the state your baby is in, you get to know your baby better and know how best to respond and when it is the best time to play, feed, or let him sleep. According to Chitty et al (2007) there are six main states:

Deep Sleep

This state is very important for your baby as he grows the most. In this state, your baby's eyes are closed, he lies still; his breathing is steady and regular and he is hard to rouse. It is imperative to allow your baby to be left undisturbed during this time. So do not wake baby up to feed or play.

Light Sleep

In this state, your baby's eyes are closed. You may notice that your baby's eyes flutter under the his eyelids. This is known as rapid eye movements (REM). He may show some body or facial movements and is easy to rouse. He may display some sucking or smiling movements or whine. However, this does not necessarily mean that your baby is hungry.

Drowsy/Dozing

In this state your baby is half awake. His eyes are open, but he remains drowsy. As your baby is not fully awake, he may fall back to sleep again. Therefore allow your baby to fully awake by himself.

Quiet Alert

This is the best state to perform any activity with your baby. In this state, your baby's eyes are wide and his face is bright and he may be slightly active. He will feed best in this state and enjoy play, and may like a massage. However, babies have a short attention span, so be careful not to overwhelm your baby and incorporate periods of rest during any activity. The key is to pace your baby.

Active Alert

In this state, your baby is very active. He is more responsive to sound and this may be a good time to feed your baby especially at night. You may want to offer your baby a feed as your baby may be hungry. If your baby is fretful, you could try slowing down or giving your baby a break from any activity you are undertaking.

TUNE IN TO YOUR BABY

Crying

This is the easiest state to identify. Your baby cries to let you know that he needs a break from whatever you are doing. You may calm your baby by trying some of the following: using a soothing rhythmic approach such as rocking, stroking your baby's back or head. Talking to your baby alerts him that you are trying to get to identify the cause of your baby's distress. Singing softly to your baby can help soothe him. Hold your baby close to you on your chest so that he can feel your heart beating and this may calm him down. If this does not work, take him out for walk, or a ride in the buggy or car. Your baby may calm down to some 'white noise' such as the vacuum cleaner, washing machine or dishwasher. It may remind your baby of life in the womb and calm him down. Sometimes your baby will calm down best without any help and self-soothe. He may do this by sucking on his fingers, fist, or tongue, bringing his hands to his mouth, changing how he is laying or looking and listening to faces and voices.

Remember that crying is the main way that a baby communicates his needs. A baby will cry when he is tired, hungry, cold, hot, sick, bored, scared, lonely – whenever he is not comfortable. But don't worry, be patient. Eventually, you will be able to interpret your baby's cry. As you do, your baby will learn to trust you knowing that you understand him and know his needs.

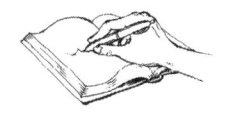

Please turn to the appendix and look for the heading *Your Baby States*.

Containment

When a baby is distressed, it is important for parents to be able to contain their baby's emotions. Containment is a theory that was developed by Wilfred Bion, a British psychoanalyst. The idea is that we unconsciously project an aspect of ourselves onto someone else, either to get rid of it or as way of communicating a particularly painful or difficult feeling. It is the notion of another person being able to hold on to these feelings, and then give them back having detoxified them, making it bearable. This relies on the person doing the containing having a certain amount of self-knowledge and the ability to know what is theirs and what is someone else's. Let me illustrate this. When a baby is born, he may be anxious about the fact that his world has changed. He may get overwhelmed about the new situation of things. He cannot express himself using language. So he cries. The mum tries to guess what the problem may be, but gets it wrong. Baby gets frustrated, and cries even more. Mum gets anxious and her heart rate gets faster. As she is holding baby, she projects her anxiety onto baby. He picks up the fact that his mum is now anxious too because he can hear her heart beating faster. He cries even more and the cycle continues. In this example, the mum has taken the baby's feelings and they have become – she is thus unable to contain her baby.

When a mum is able to contain her infant, it means that she can grasp her baby's anxieties, and process his emotional experience and state of mind, without being overwhelmed by it; taking the panic out of the child's anxiety. In time the infant will begin to learn about his mum's ability to handle anxiety, and will eventually be able to deal with anxiety and frustration without his mum's intervention.

A mum contains her baby's anxiety and emotions by keeping her baby in mind. She does this by *stepping into baby's shoes* and imagining what her baby is feeling but not taking his problem on. She will be like a container for her baby and the child will respond to her. This is important because if a person seeks containment from someone who is not able to give it, at best he ends up feeling no better. But it can leave him feeling worse or even more overwhelmed as demonstrated in the example above.

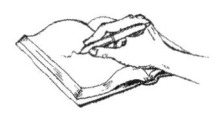

Please turn to the appendix and look for the heading *Contain Your Baby's Emotions.*

Bonding and Attachment

Bonding is the process by which a new parent develops a deep affection and protective love for their baby. It is a unique emotional relationship between you and your baby. It is what makes you as a parent, do whatever you need to do to protect and nurture your little one. It is what makes you sacrifice your own needs to ensure that your baby's needs are met. Bonding helps your baby feel secure. Through the strong bond that you as a parent have for your baby, he learns to form other relationships.

Whereas a parent bonds with their infant, a baby attaches to his primary caregiver (often the mother). Attachment describes the enduring connection that develops between a baby and his main caregiver. This is characterised by a tendency to seek and maintain closeness to the caregiver, especially during stressful situations (Bowlby, 1988). As a mum when you are reliably responding to your baby's needs, it forms the basis for a secure attachment. It teaches your baby to trust you, to communicate their feelings to you, and eventually to trust others as well. As you and your baby connect with one r baby learns how to have a healthy sense of self be in a loving, empathic relationship. Thus, it is vital u as a mum to try to bond with your infant prior to his birth as this will enable your baby to further develop this bond after birth and enable the baby to become securely attached to you (Robinson et al, 2012).

Most babies are born ready to connect to their parents. However, some babies may have problems that can get in the way of secure attachment and bonding. These include: babies that experienced problems in the womb, or at the time of birth; premature infants that have spent time in intensive care, or babies where there is no constant caregiver. At other times the problems with bonding is on the part of the parents. Parents who themselves did not experience a secure attachment when they were infants may have trouble emotionally connecting with their babies. Other things that may affect your ability to bond with your baby include: depression, anxiety, or other emotional problems; high levels of stress, living in an unsafe environment, drug or alcohol problems, and abuse or neglect in childhood (Robinson et al, 2012). Having any of the above problems does not mean you will not be able to eventually bond with your baby. The sooner the problems are identified, the easier they are to correct. Thus, if you or your baby encounter any of the above problems, it is important to get support from your paediatrician, General Practitioner or family doctor, Health visitor or someone trained in early intervention.

Breast-feeding

Breast-feeding is the healthiest way to feed your baby. It benefits both yourself and your baby. Breast-feeding is the healthiest choice for you because it reduces your risk later in life of pre-menopausal breast cancer, ovarian cancer, and bone fractures from osteoporosis. It is convenient as you don't have to wash or sterilise bottles or prepare feeds. Your

TUNE IN TO YOUR BABY

baby's feeds are ready made with each feed made to meet baby's needs. For your baby, breast-feeding helps your baby's immunity and helps protect against illnesses such as tummy bugs (gastroenteritis), colds, ear and urinary infections. Breast milk also helps to protect your baby against serious illnesses, such as childhood diabetes and leukaemia. breast milk has long-chain polyunsaturated fatty acids, which are essential for helping your baby's brain develop. Exclusively breast-feeding for the first few months can improve your baby's cognitive development. In theory, this means that breast-feeding your baby could make him more intelligent. Breast-feeding reduces the risk of cot death. It also helps build a strong bond between you and your baby, both physically and emotionally. You and your baby will enjoy it, and you will feel a real sense of achievement to see him growing and developing. And it will be all down to you. All you need to do is eat well, keep hydrated and have plenty of rest.

Your breast milk is designed for your baby and contains everything your baby needs for around the first six months of life. However, like any new skill it is not easy and takes a great deal of time and practice to work well. Immediately after the birth of your baby, you are ready to breastfeed. Your breasts contain colostrum, which is very concentrated, and as such your baby requires only a small amount at each feed. Colostrum is full of antibodies that help protect your baby against infections that you have had in the past. The first few feeds help 'line' your baby's gut protecting him from germs and reducing the chances of him getting allergic conditions such as asthma and eczema later in life. As well as the antibodies already in your breast milk, your body will make new antibodies as soon as you are exposed to an infection, which affords baby extra protection against getting the infection from you.

Once your baby is born, try to have skin-to-skin contact straight after birth. If there are no complications of pregnancy and birth, babies are often very alert in the first hour. Babies that have been placed on their mothers belly immediately after delivery have been known to crawl to their mum's nipple, latch on and suckle. If you require assistance with breast-feeding, ask your midwife to help you. As discussed in the previous chapter, breast-feeding, like any other skill can be hard work in the early days. As such it is important to prepare your mind for the challenges breast-feeding can bring.

When a woman initiates breast-feeding, she may be unsure about what to do, and worry about whether the baby is latching on properly or if the baby is getting enough milk. The frequency of feeds that a newborn requires may also cause a mum to believe that her infant is not getting enough. It is thus important to highlight a few points as this can give you the confidence and assurance required to continue breast-feeding if you are feeling like giving up in the early days. When your baby was in your womb, he was continuously fed via the placenta and never felt hungry. When a baby is born, he becomes hungry and requires milk from his mother. The baby has a very small stomach, the size of a walnut and only has a capacity for about 30mls of milk (1 ounce). Therefore, when baby feeds and fills his stomach, he is satisfied and stops suckling except for comfort. Within an hour or so, his stomach is empty and he requires another feed. This is the usual routine in the first few days. But over time, as the baby matures, his stomach grows bigger and he is thus able to take more breast milk and have longer intervals between feeds.

Another reason that some women give up breast-feeding in the early days is due to baby's initial weight loss. However, babies do not lose weight because they are breast-fed, but because they are fed! As was explained earlier in this chapter, a baby does not use his gut whilst in the womb. His gut is lined with meconium (a dark, tar-like substance) to keep it from collapsing on itself. After a baby is born, once he starts to ingest milk, this produces a laxative effect and the baby is purged of the meconium. The meconium is dense, sticky and

TUNE IN TO YOUR BABY

quite heavy which is why a baby loses weight in the first few days. Babies can lose up to 10 per cent of their birth weight but will usually regain their birth weight in the first two weeks of life.

You may still be wondering how you will know that your baby is getting enough milk. If you have latched baby on to the breast properly, your nipples should not hurt, although the first few sucks may feel strong. Your baby should have a large mouthful of breast. His chin should be firmly touching your breast. Your baby's cheeks should stay rounded whilst suckling. He should rhythmically take long sucks and swallow, pausing intermittently; and come off the breast on his own when he finishes the feed. If you still require support with breast-feeding let your midwife know. There are often breast-feeding support groups in the community or a breast-feeding support adviser may be able to visit you at home.

> *'What good mothers and fathers instinctively feel like doing for their babies is usually best after all.'*
> Benjamin Spock, Paediatrician

You may want to know how often your baby should be breast-fed. The answer to this is that baby will let you know. Baby-led feeding! Your baby will let you know that he is ready for feeding by giving you feeding cues. Most babies will 'ask politely' in the first instance by moving their eyes rapidly, putting their fingers into their mouth, rooting (opening their mouth as though they were about to breastfeed) and becoming restless (The Baby Friendly Initiative, 2011). This is a much easier time to feed than when he has got to the stage of crying and these subtle cues are much easier to pick up when your baby is close by. It is thus important to keep him close to you so that you can recognise his feeding cues. Following these feeding cues works better than waiting a set number of hours before attempting each feeding. Further, trying to wake a baby from a deep sleep will prove frustrating for both of you. However, as a general rule, until breast-feeding is well established, you can expect that your baby will feed *at least* 6-8 times in each 24-hour period although it may be more frequent.

Night feeds are important when establishing breast-feeding as prolactin levels are at their highest. Prolactin is the hormone responsible for helping the alveolar cells in the breast to make breast milk, and it is released from the pituitary gland in response to a suckling baby. There is evidence that the level of prolactin in the milk is higher during times of highest milk production and that the highest prolactin levels occur in the middle of the night between 2:00 am and 6:00 am (Mohrbacher and Stock, 2003). Therefore, although it may be harder to feed at night, it is important to breastfeed during the night to maintain your breast milk supply.

Whilst breast-feeding, there is no need to give other fluids, even water. Breast milk is produced on a demand and supply basis. Thus the more you breastfeed, the more milk is produced. If your baby feels hungrier, just offer more feeds. This can happen especially when your baby has a growth spurt. Babies grow the most outside the womb in the first year of life. By the time your baby is one year old, he will be about three times his birth weight. He will have several growth spurts in the first year of life usually occurring at 7–10 days old, about three weeks, followed by 6 weeks, 3 months, 6 months and 9 months. These ages are all approximate and babies may have a growth spurt at other times as well. As long as baby is growing appropriately and is healthy, a growth spurt at any age should not be cause for concern and they usually last for about 2-3 days.

There are other reasons why a mum may find breast-feeding challenging. These include engorgement, blocked ducts and mastitis. It is important to keep the milk flowing. Therefore, gently massage the affected area and breastfeed as often as you can. Drink plenty of fluids and get sufficient rest to promote healing. Sometimes, due to the use of antibiotics, thrush may develop. If this happens, you may notice you may suddenly get sore nipples after several weeks of pain-free breast-feeding. You also could have achy breasts or shooting pains deep in the breast during or after feedings. It is important to see your doctor or health visitor who can confirm if it is thrush and prescribe anti-fungal treatment for you and your baby. Be sure to complete the course of treatment. Whilst breast-feeding, it is important to wear a comfortable, well-fitting supportive bra as some of the above problems may be as a result of wearing tight bras.

Some babies are born with a tongue-tie – a tight piece of skin between the underside of the tongue and the floor of their mouth. This can affect feeding, creating difficulty for your baby in latching on to the breast. Tongue-tie may require a procedure to loosen it. Therefore if you have concerns speak with your midwife or health visitor.

Despite wanting to breastfeed, there are times when a woman is unable to. This includes maternal-infant separation either due to illness on the part of the mother, infant or both. If this happens inform your doctors about your wishes to breastfeed. If it is your infant that is unwell, you can still breastfeed by expressing breast milk and baby can be fed your milk through a tube. There are often breast-feeding advisers in most maternity units who can assist with this.

Some women may want to express breast milk and give it through a bottle. This is fine. However, if your baby is able to breastfeed, it is best to wait until breast-feeding is established to avoid nipple confusion. In the early days, it is easier for a baby to suck from a bottle than to suckle from the breast. By about four weeks, breast-feeding should be established and you can offer one or two feeds of expressed breast milk through a bottle so that others can get involved in feeding your baby. However, it is important to continue to put baby to the breast because a breast pump is not as effective at drawing out breast milk, as a baby's jaw.

It is also important not to compare the volume of breast milk with that of artificial formula. One ounce of breast milk is not equal to one ounce of formula. Breast milk composition changes with each feed. The way the baby suckles at the breast determines the constitution of the milk your baby gets. If he is thirsty, the milk is adjusted to quench his thirst. If he is very hungry, breast milk composition changes to meet that need. Hence, the uniqueness of breast milk and its production. Your baby gets each meal to order!

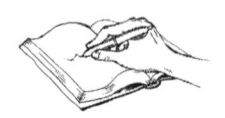

Please turn to the appendix and look for the heading *Breast-feeding Your Baby – How is it Going?*

Sleep

As a new mother, you may wonder how much sleep your baby needs as he appears to be sleeping all the time. A newborn baby is constantly growing and as such requires more sleep than an adult. A newborn baby requires enough and good, quality sleep for proper brain development. When sleeping, a baby dreams most of the time. Research evidence shows that dreaming stimulates a baby's brain and thus assists in its healthy development. Good sleep as a child also promotes general health and well-being. The first six months are crucial for developing good sleeping habits, as it is in these months that baby's sleep patterns mature most quickly and the stage is set for sleep through life.

A newborn baby should sleep on average for about 16 hours daily with three naps during the day. From one to three months of age, your baby should sleep up to 15 hours daily sleeping longer at night as they age. From six to twelve months, babies have about two naps a day and can sleep up to 14 hours daily. However, it is important to remember that your baby is unique and as such may require more or less sleep. It is important to note that your baby may not sleep through the night and may wake up to feed before he settles back to sleep.

A baby has no set routine straight after birth and needs to be taught. However, it is best to wait until breast-feeding has been established before trying to set up a sleep routine. By the time your baby is about three months old is a good time to start to follow a set pattern every night. This could include: bathing, changing into bed clothes, reading a bedtime story, cuddling, turning the lights down, etc. In this way baby will know that it is time to wind down and get ready for sleep. By about six months, your baby may be ready to sleep through the night.

> *'Nothing is particularly hard if you divide it into small jobs.'*
> Henry Ford, American industrialist

Understanding What Your Baby Needs – Maslow's Hierarchy of Needs

An easy way to understand what a baby might need and then try to meet them is to take a look at Maslow's hierarchy of needs. Abraham Maslow set out five fundamental human needs that are hierarchical in nature. The lower the needs in the hierarchy, the more essential they are and the more a person will tend to abandon the higher needs in order to adequately meet the lower needs. Maslow believed that various needs had to be met for an individual to feel complete, with physiological needs at the base, followed by safety needs and social needs.

The five needs are:

1. **Physiological**: oxygen, water, food, shelter and sleep, etc.
2. **Safety**: security, stability, protection from physical and emotional harm.
3. **Love and belonging**: affection, belonging, acceptance, friendship, community.
4. **Esteem**: Divided into internal ones – the need for self-respect, confidence, autonomy and achievement and external ones – the need for the respect of others, status, fame, recognition and attention.
5. **Self-actualisation**: doing that which maximises one's potential and fulfils one's innate aspirations.

I need to be free
Give me independence

I need to feel good about myself
Let me explore safely

I need to be loved and to belong
Show you care. Love me abundantly

I need to feel safe
Protect me. Help me feel safe and secure

I need to survive outside the womb
Feed me, keep me warm, let me breathe and let me sleep

INDEPENDENCE ↕ DEPENDENCE

Baby's Needs – Maslow's Hierarchy of Needs

When a baby is first born, his main needs are physiological. He needs to survive outside the womb and requires oxygen, food, warmth, and sleep. His main priority is survival. At first, your baby does not know if you will be able to provide these needs for him. But he is dependent on you. So he communicates these needs to you by crying. As you respond to him and begin to meet his needs, he begins to get to know you and develop trust in you. He sends you a cue; you read the cue well and respond to it, he trusts you. Over and over again, this cycle is repeated and the baby starts to feel safe and develops confidence and trust in you.

Then the baby moves to the next hierarchy. The baby is now safe and trusts you, but wants more than that and starts to love you. This love is based on trust. You have met baby's needs and kept baby safe and secure and now he loves you and expresses this love. When he sees strangers he is wary: he does not know and love them. As a result, he does not want to be separated from you. He feels securely attached to you. As time goes on baby moves to the next phase and starts to feel good about himself. Through trial and error, he starts to learn that he can learn to depend on himself some more. He begins to move, crawl and eventually learns to walk. He is now free and wants to explore the world. You try to set him boundaries but he does not like your rules. So he breaks them. According to your baby his newfound freedom allows him some independence. In order words, he says to himself that he has been dependent on you for so long and he now needs to be free of you.

As highlighted above, Maslow's hierarchy of needs stresses that the basic needs of a baby such as physiological needs which include nutrition, rest and activity must be met in order for the child to progress. By understanding your baby you can fulfil his needs and it will enable him to move up the hierarchy.

Love

The importance of love for a baby cannot be overemphasised. Love is essential for the proper development of the baby's brain. When a baby is shown love, he attaches himself securely to his main caregiver and it serves as a template for other relationships he will form. It is also essential to love yourself and take care of yourself. You will only be able to meet your baby's needs when you look after yourself. Therefore, ensure that you eat well, stay hydrated and get plenty of sleep. Your baby needs you to be fit and well. Also, when a mum loves herself, she demonstrates this love and the child learns to love himself too. (How to love yourself will be discussed in more detail in the next chapter). Finally, it is important to show love for the significant others in your life – your partner, family and friends as your baby will use the way you relate to those you love as a template for forming other relationships.

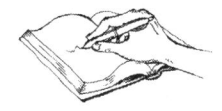

> Please turn to the appendix and look for the heading *Love for You, Baby and Others*.

Learning Through Play

Play is essential for your baby's social, emotional, physical, and cognitive development. It's your baby's way of learning about his body and the environment. He has five senses and he will employ them all as he tries to discover the world around him, especially in the first year. Your baby is very inquisitive and is curious about his surroundings. He is continuously asking himself what things feel like, sound, taste like. Your baby will explore his environment as this is how he learns about it. He will experiment with things – his toys, clothes, food, etc. Therefore allow opportunities for messy play and for your child to explore his surroundings safely.

In the first year of life, babies learn through social play, interacting with you and others around them. They love to smile, look, and laugh. Therefore allow plenty of opportunities to play with your child. Even a newborn baby will try to copy what you do such as blinking when you blink or sticking his tongue out in imitation of you. You can progress to tickles and blowing raspberries on his belly to invoke a smile. As your baby matures, he may enjoy nursery rhymes interactive games such as peek-a-boo, pat-a-cake and round-and-round-the-garden. You may want to attend local playgroups where your child can learn to interact with other babies and children.

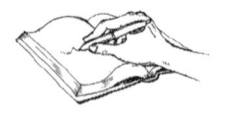

Please turn to the appendix and look for the heading *Playing with Your Baby*.

> *'Success for me is to raise happy, healthy human beings.'*
> Kelly LeBrock, Actress and model

I'm a Mum!

Becoming a mum is a hugely rewarding experience, but it can also be challenging. In the first few days and weeks, it can be quite exhausting as all the baby appears to do is to take from you. However, as the baby begins to mature, he starts to give back, from a smile, to a kiss and a cuddle. It is important to celebrate what is good about your new role. As a mother, you will probably make lots of new friendships with other mothers and can look forward to your children growing up together. In some societies, becoming a mum improves your status as it proves that you are fertile and have given birth to a child to prove it.

According to Ellison (2005), motherhood expands the mind, boosting brain power and making a woman smarter. She states that this happens in five areas: perception, efficiency, resilience, motivation, and emotional intelligence. Perception, deals primarily with the five senses. Research has demonstrated that pregnant women had sharper vision, noticing a lot more, than women who weren't expecting a baby. Pregnant women also have an enhanced sense of smell, which theoretically serves to protect the unborn baby from things that may be harmful such as cigarette smoke. Other studies have shown that mothers can experience a boost in motivation, courage, and the ability to multitask and cope with stress. Evidence suggests that oxytocin - the labour and breast feeding hormone, improves a mum's memory and capacity for learning. One of the biggest brain boosts for mothers is emotional intelligence - the ability to see the world through someone else's eyes. Whilst you can walk away from a person you disagree with, if you don't agree with your child, you can't walk away. Instead, you do whatever you have to do to understand the way he sees things.

Whatever reasons you have for celebrating this new role, enjoy them, as it will help you cope with the challenges. It is also essential to be happy in your new role. If you are not, baby will pick up on this and may get anxious. Therefore, think happy thoughts so you can feel happy and be happy. Prior to the birth of your baby, you imagined life as a new mother. Try to make a list now of the benefits and drawbacks of motherhood and compare it with your previous list.

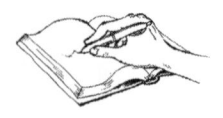

Please turn to the appendix and look for the heading *How Do I Feel about Being a Mum? – Motherhood Gains and Losses.*

Many challenges come with your new role. Loss of your independence, tiredness and lack of sleep, loss of your identity, loss of friendships, etc. It is important that you learn to adjust to your new role and handle the challenges that come with it. A good way to do this is to set goals. Set goals about where you are now and where you want to go. Map out your parenting journey. Benjamin Franklin's famous quote states that: 'if you fail to plan, you plan to fail'. Therefore plan how you will deal with the challenges parenting brings making a list of whose help you will enlist. Draw up an action plan and review it periodically. Take responsibility and track your progress. Your confidence will grow through action.

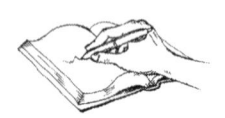

Please turn to the appendix and look for the heading *How does it feel to be a Mum?*

Motherhood: It's all Learning and Growing

As a mother, you are your baby's new teacher, but you are also a student. You are a new parent and thus will learn a great deal about your baby and yourself, others that you love and your new role. As you cope with the challenges that motherhood brings you will grow in confidence and learn resilience. Commit to enjoying your new baby and your new role. View everyday as a learning experience. Be willing to learn in order to enable you to grow in to your new role. Remember that it's a role where you learn on the job. Your CV will grow as you do. Most importantly you're not allowed to quit. So, be determined to enjoy it!

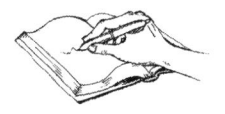

Please turn to the appendix and look for the heading *Celebrate Motherhood! It's all About Learning and Growing.*

Sharing My Learning

- Try to step into your baby's shoes and see things through their eyes. Start by imagining your baby's journey to the world during labour and childbirth. Then you will understand the rationale for his behaviour and help him adjust to life outside the womb.

- In the early days, life outside the womb is hard for your baby. Try to recreate the conditions baby is used to outside the womb. Give lots of cuddles and skin-to-skin contact.

- Pay close attention to your baby's responses. Use his senses.

- You are your baby's teacher. Whatever you want your baby to do, do lots of it. If you want your baby to smile, smile a lot. If you want your baby to love, show him lots of love.

- Observe your baby's cues and states, and respond to them. The more you do, the more your baby will develop trust in you and your ability to care for him.

- Contain your baby's emotions but don't take his emotions on.

- Bond well with your baby, and baby should become securely attached to you.

- Prepare your mind to breastfeed. Breast-feeding is beneficial for you and baby. Although it can be challenging in the early days, breast-feeding eventually gets easier over time. If you require support to breastfeed or express breast milk, ask for it.

- In the early days, baby's main need is for survival, then safety, then love and belonging, esteem and eventually some independence.

- You are baby's best playmate!
- Celebrate being a mother, and prepare for the challenges it brings.
- Commit to enjoying every day in your new role.
- Being a mum is all about learning and growing!

> *'Love means to commit yourself without guarantee.'*
> Anne Campbell, Politician

Chapter 4
Wow! No One Said It Would Be This Hard

This is how I felt when Joshua was a few weeks old. Hence, the reason for the title of this chapter. The honeymoon period of being a new mum had passed and all I seemed to focus on was how my life was now in comparison to how my life could have been or should be. I loved Joshua but somehow didn't feel as ecstatic as I felt when I initially had him. I felt I had lost my sense of identity. As I was now a mother, I was not referred to by my first name but as *Mama Joshua* (Mum of Joshua). This is the custom in the Yoruba part of Nigeria where I originate from. Many Yoruba women are proud to be identified by their children as this is a celebration of motherhood and a symbol of fertility. However, as I was mourning the loss of myself, and craving my life before I had Joshua, I did not want my main identity to be around my son, despite being proud to have him. I felt I should be myself first, before being Joshua's mother. I also felt a loss of control as my extended family thought they knew better what I should do for my son. Every one of them appeared to have some advice about what I should do for Joshua and I found this so frustrating. Therefore in this chapter I will focus on how you can manage some challenging situations you may encounter as you strive to raise your infant.

I will also discuss the myth of 'perfect' parenting and discuss strategies that can help you manage yourself and enable you to tune in to your baby and enjoy parenting.

You have had your baby and probably feel as I did. The feelings of excitement that you once had are starting to wane. Your partner has gone back to work. Your family and friends have celebrated the birth of your baby with you and have returned to their normal business. Suddenly you feel alone and stuck with your baby who you love very dearly. You have a deep feeling of loss of self and uncertainty. You adore your baby and he excites you. But your emotions appear to rollercoaster between happiness, confusion, fear, and occasionally resentment. These feelings can make you feel ashamed, guilty and alone as you think they are not right. Again, I must stress that you are not alone. Many women experience these feelings, although most do not understand why they happen. These feelings are often referred to as 'motherhood blues' and are natural and not to be confused with postnatal depression which is more incapacitating. You can liken the feelings in motherhood to a scale, where excitement and delight exist on one end and postnatal depression on the other. Motherhood blues exists somewhere between both ends of the scale. They are a part of the grieving process that occurs when the realisation hits you that your life before you had a baby will not be the same again. You mourn the loss of yourself, your identity and independence. You also realise that being a parent is hard work and as you strive to be perfect at it you realise that you are far from perfection. Let me start by putting you out of your misery.

> *'24/7. Once you sign on to be a mother, that's the only shift they offer.'*
> Jodi Picoult, Author

Practice Doesn't Make Perfect!

Prior to the birth of your baby you probably always dreamed that you will be a perfect parent. You probably imagined how life with a child would be and all the things you will do with your baby. Now, all that you dreamed about has not come true and this makes you feel low. According to Demartini, 'many mothers experience feelings of emptiness, loss of identity and then anger and resentment when their fantasy of motherhood does not match up to the reality – when they realise that motherhood is more about sleepless nights, screaming babies and dirty nappies than blissful bonding moments between a calm mum and her angelic baby.' This is worsened by what you observe and hear. You see other mothers who appear to have bonded with their babies and look to be enjoying their new roles. They look like perfect mothers. You speak with them and all they talk about is how they are enjoying motherhood. But there is reason behind this. In her article, *The Motherhood Blues*, Camilla Rankin states that 'mothers rarely talk about the deeper sense of self-loss, confusion or anger they have about motherhood.' As mothers we often keep these negative feelings to ourselves because we are conditioned to believe that becoming a mum is the best thing that could happen to us. However, when it comes to parenting, there is no such thing as perfection. Furthermore, children do not need perfect parents! You can confirm that even your parents were not perfect because you could easily pick out their flaws. As you grew up, you probably compared them with other parents who in your opinion were better than them. Your child will probably do the same as he grows and will let you know how far from perfection you are, as a parent. Therefore, accept it! Perfect parents don't exist. Well, not on planet earth.

What does exist, however, is good-enough parenting. Good-enough parents are able to tune in to their child, and are responsive to his needs, particularly emotionally, resulting in the child's sense of being understood, cared for and valued. To tune in to one's child, a parent seeks to understand the child's perspective and his needs, even though they cannot always voice this (Peterson, 1999).

Although parenting can be challenging, make it your goal to tune in as much as possible to the needs of your child. Over time you will without doubt grow in knowledge about your child. Like any other role we may have in life, at first we often learn how not to do, before we learn how to do. The same is true with parenting. As parents we will naturally fail at times. If at first you do not succeed, sooner or later you will come to better understand your child and better able to meet his emerging needs. If you are committed to parenting as an important job, you will correct errors made and learn from the experience. Therefore, do not be afraid to make mistakes as a parent, as you will learn from them. With practice, you will become better at parenting. You will be able to trust and reflect on your actions and resolve mistakes as they occur. As you do so, the bond between you and your child will be strengthened. For that reason, embrace being a good *enough* parent. Do not put unnecessary pressure on yourself trying to strive for perfection. It is an illusion, and you may be setting yourself up to fail.

Parenting is Learning

There are four states of consciousness and competence that a person may pass through when learning a new skill. Knowing this can help you to manage your emotions during the sometimes daunting learning process of parenting. (See The Circle of Learning diagram).

1. Unconscious Incompetence

At this stage a person does not understand or know how to do something and does not necessarily recognise the deficit. In other words, **you don't know**

that you don't know. At this level, ignorance is bliss and you may well be happily naive, not realising that you are not competent and have a complete lack of knowledge and skills. Even though you may be confident, it is not based on your abilities.

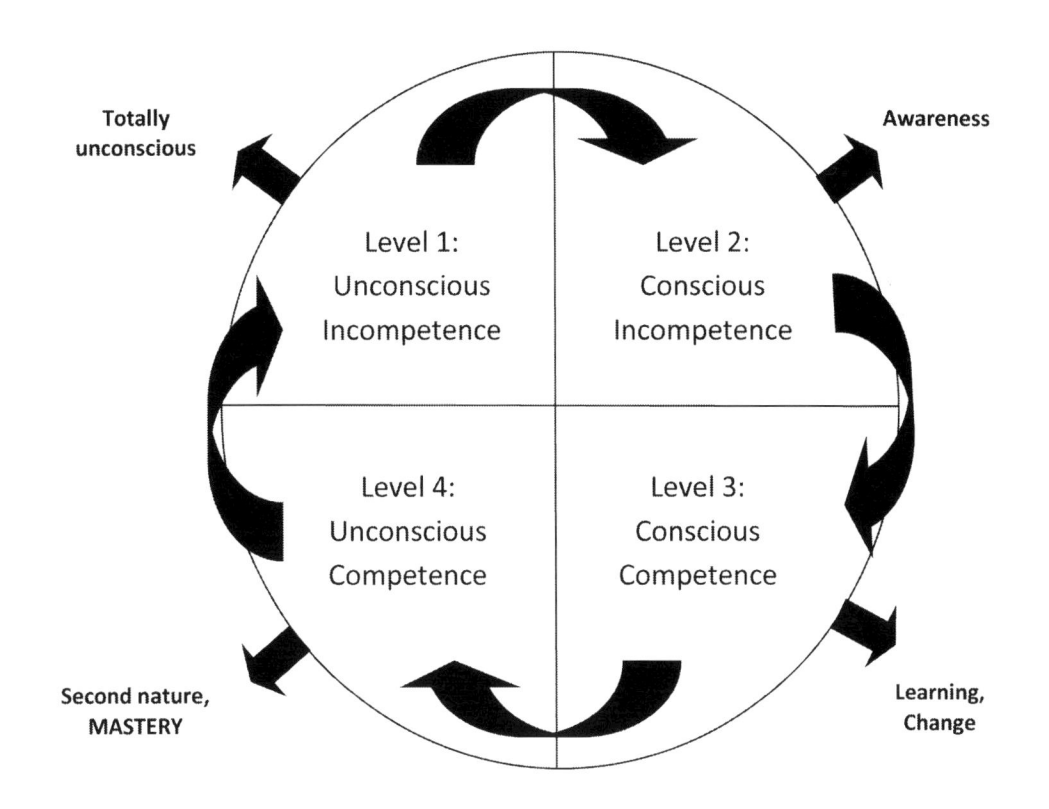

```
                    Totally unconscious
                           ↑
        ┌──────────────────┼──────────────────┐
        │   Level 1:       │   Level 2:       │
        │   Unconscious    │   Conscious      │
        │   Incompetence   │   Incompetence   │
        ├──────────────────┼──────────────────┤
        │   Level 4:       │   Level 3:       │
        │   Unconscious    │   Conscious      │
        │   Competence     │   Competence     │
        └──────────────────┴──────────────────┘
     Second nature,                      Learning,
     MASTERY                             Change
                           ↓
                       Awareness
```

The Circle of Learning

2. Conscious Incompetence

Though you don't know how to do something, you recognise the deficit, as well as the value of a new skill in addressing the deficit. **You know that you don't know**. At this level you find that there are skills you need to learn, and you may be shocked to discover that there are others who are much more competent than you. As you realise that your ability is limited, your confidence drops. You realise that you are not as expert as perhaps you thought you were or thought you could be; and may go through an uncomfortable period as you learn these new skills.

3. Conscious Competence

At this level, you know how to do something. However, demonstrating the skill or knowledge requires concentration. You may break it down into steps, and there is heavy conscious involvement in executing the new skill. **You know that you know**. But work on refining them. As you get more practice and experience, these become increasingly automatic.

4. Unconscious Competence

At this level your new skills become habits, and you perform the task effortlessly and with automatic ease. You have had so much practice that it has become 'second nature' and can be performed easily. You no longer have to think about what you are doing, **you don't know that you know**.

In order to learn to parent and become an expert at parenting your child, you will move through the four stages of the ladder. You will become conscious of what you do and do not know and eventually become competent through the learning experience. For example, at first you may not know much about breast-feeding your infant and not know that you don't know. Eventually, you have your baby and realise that you know very little about breast-feeding and you observe other women breast-feeding their infants with ease. Someone asks you if your baby is latching on well. You ask what that means. This sudden realisation about your deficit in knowledge can leave you overwhelmed and make you want to give up. This is often where lots of mistakes are made as you are still not competent. However, as stated earlier we often learn first how not to do, before we learn how to do. Therefore, making mistakes can be central to the learning process. In time, you will move to the conscious competence stage where you are competent but still thinking about what you are doing. At this stage breast-feeding may seem like a procedure, and you are carefully thinking the steps through. Sooner or later, you will move into the unconscious competent stage, when you have mastered the art of breast-feeding and can breastfeed with your eyes closed, effortlessly. Problem solved you may think! True. But with parenting there are many skills to learn. Hence, once a skill is learned, you almost immediately need to learn another. You now know how to breastfeed your baby and do so effortlessly for six months and then you have to wean your baby. You are now at level one again (unconscious incompetence). You don't know what you don't know! Thus, as a parent, learning is a continuous experience. As your baby grows, there are new experiences and new problems and the cycle begins again.

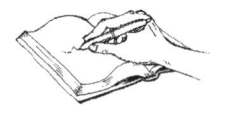

Please turn to the appendix and look for the heading *Where are You in The Learning Circle?*

Making Decisions? Remember, It's *Your* Baby!

A source of anxiety after you have had a baby may be when others that you care about other than your partner consider your baby theirs and try to parent your child. It may be your parents, your partner's parents, your siblings, your partner's siblings, friends or other family members. As your baby grows they tell you what to do. This is often not a problem if you are in agreement with their advice. However, this can be a potential source of conflict, when their advice contradicts what you want to do. Sometimes, you may find yourself making choices that are not based on what you think, but what others would do. I discuss below a useful theory that can help you to make decisions and stick to them.

Transactional Analysis

Transactional Analysis was first described by Eric Berne, a psychoanalyst, in the 1950s. It is the analysis of communication patterns that we set up with other people and ourselves. It aspires to the philosophy that everyone is all right and people should be accepted for who they are and not for what they do. From early in life we unconsciously make decisions as to how we will be and behave in the world. As children, when we made decisions about how to behave, we did so with reference to how we felt the adults around us wanted us to act. These were guesses and were not always right. Unfortunately, we grow up with this pattern of behaviour and continue to act in like manner even though we are now adult. Therefore, it is useful for us to sort out our thoughts so we can keep the part that serves us in our lives and change the part that does not. By using transactional analysis, we can bring these old decisions into our awareness, understand why we made them and make age-appropriate decisions. Berne identified that we transact or communicate in three main ways which he called 'ego states' – Parent, Adult and Child.

Parent Ego State

The Parent ego state describes thoughts, feelings, and behaviours that are learned from our parents or other caretakers. It is demonstrated in two ways - the Nurturing Parent, which is the soft, caring and loving side; and the Critical Parent, the part that tries to make the child act as the parent wants. You will recognise when you are in this state when you use words like 'should', 'ought', and 'need'. Whilst some advice from others is useful, advice that aims to take control away from you and take away your ability to be yourself and decide on your behaviour as an adult is restricting and unhelpful.

Adult Ego State

The Adult ego state is based on reality – the here and now. It is the part of our personality that is accurate, and sees, hears, thinks, and can come up with solutions to problems based on the facts and not out-dated messages from the past. Choice is the most useful word to hold in your head in this state. Adult thinking relies on you saying 'I can weigh up the benefits and drawbacks and make a decision on my reality and circumstances'.

> *'Aim for success not perfection.'*
> Dr David Burns, Psychiatrist and author

Child Ego State

In this state, there are three ways of behaving. The first is the Adapted Child. In this state you do whatever someone wants you to do and not really what you want to do. The second is the Rebellious Child, when you rebel against any advice given for the sake of it. The third one is the Free Child that loves spontaneity. It is the side of us that experiences the world in a direct and immediate way.

It is possible to determine what ego state you or those around you are using. You can do this by observing the tone of voice and words used, body language, and emotions displayed. A person adopting the Nurturing Parent ego state often uses a soothing tone of voice whilst the Critical Parent ego state employs a harsh or critical tone. When in the Adult ego state, the tone is even and clear (Solomon, 2003).

Making Decisions as a Parent – Be Adult About It!

As a parent it is important to make adult decisions – based on the present and on facts. Over the course of your life as a parent you will have to make countless decisions. How should I feed my baby? What should I name him? Should I go back to work? Should I work full-time or part-time? What about childcare – nanny, nursery or childminder? And many others. Rather than feeling you ought to do something for example, breastfeed your baby, it is important that you consider all the information available to you, weighing the pros and cons of each option that you have and make a decision based on them. If you have a partner, jointly discuss and come to an agreement. Once you do, you do not owe anyone an explanation for your decision. Those who love you should eventually respect your decision even if they don't agree with it. Even if you later find out that the decision you initially made is no longer right for you, just make another decision – decide on another action.

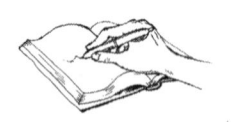

Please turn to the Appendix and look for the heading *Making Adult Decisions – Weighing up the Pros and Cons.*

Your Baby is Unique – Don't Compare!

It's human nature to want to compare your child with other children. However, this can cause you a lot of anxiety. Remember that your baby is special and unique. There is no other child like yours. So don't compare. When other parents try to compare their children with yours, resist the urge to turn parenting into a competition because it will rob you of the joy of parenting. Surround yourself with like-minded mums that do not want to compare their children with yours. However, if you are worried about your child's development, speak with your health visitor.

Please turn to the Appendix and look for the heading *My Special Baby.*

Be Patient! View Each Day as a Learning Experience

We live in a world of instant gratification where we want things and want them now, sometimes without giving consideration to the consequences. This sometimes means that we will do anything that makes us feel better instantly but may make us feel worse in the future. Feelings take precedence over thinking and action for a quick fix. Mastering a skill is not instant and relies on delayed gratification. Parenting requires patience, work, time and practice. Although it may involve frustration, pain, discomfort and challenging feelings, choosing delayed gratification works in the long term. By so doing, you will be modelling good behaviour to your little one.

Feeding

It can be worrying for you as a mum if your baby doesn't appear to be feeding as well as you expect. It's natural to think that there is something wrong. However, most times there is nothing serious and the problem can easily be remedied. Often mothers worry that their babies vomit after every feed. If the amount is small, this is called *possetting* and happens because the band or sphincter that helps keep food in the stomach is immature. As a result, when the baby burps and brings up wind, some milk comes up too. As the baby matures, this should improve. Sometimes, the amount of milk that your baby brings up may be a lot more than a possett and this may be upsetting for you as a parent. It may be a sign that you are overfeeding your baby, so it may be worth reducing your baby's feeds and then feed him more often. It can also help if you sit him upright to enable him to keep his feeds down. Frequent vomiting may also be a symptom of gastric reflux which is easily treated. As long as your baby is gaining weight, there is usually nothing to worry about. If your baby has projectile vomit or appears to be in pain, speak with your health visitor or doctor.

Eventually your baby is about six months old and it is time to introduce solid foods. When you start weaning, the aim is to gradually introduce your baby to new tastes and textures. This is a new experience for your baby as he will have to use his tongue differently. Baby-led weaning simply means letting your baby feed himself. Initially, your baby may gag when you introduce solid foods. This sometimes causes anxiety for parents as they think their baby is going to choke. But your child will eventually learn to use his tongue in a different way to swallow thicker foods and move on to mashed or lumpier foods by seven months of age. Babies often want to be participants at meal times so give them a spoon so that they can enjoy the experience. They can also feed themselves with finger foods.

Try to expose your child to a variety of foods. Sometimes, your child may refuse foods that are offered because the taste is not pleasant. Your baby may want to vomit as he does not like the food given. However, persist with it and over time, your child will acquire a taste for the new food. Mealtimes should be fun so do not force your baby to eat. Be ready for the mess that baby will make. Babies will naturally touch and play with their food – it's all part of the learning experience. Try not to go out of your way to make separate meals for your baby. Your baby should eat what you eat as long as it is a healthy diet. Also try to eat as a family. Make mealtimes a social event.

Crying

Crying is a way that your baby shows you that he needs comfort and care. However, sometimes a baby's crying may be excessive. Excessive crying may be a sign of colic. Colic is often identified as a continuous, intense cry, angry, red flushed face, clenched fists, arched back, drawn knees and baby can't be comforted. This can leave parents feeling helpless and stressed because they are unable to comfort their infant. Although the main causes of colic remain unknown, there are several suggestions about probable causes: a build-up of wind in the gut; sensitivity to lactose – natural sugar found in milk; emotional sensitivity where baby may experience difficulty in 'turning off' his crying response. There is also evidence to show that babies with colic often have higher levels of motilin – a hormone that stimulates stomach activity (Unite/CPHVA, 2012).

If you think your baby has colic, you may want to establish a pattern by observing your baby and keeping a diary of the times your baby cries. If your baby cries for at least three hours a day, for at least three days a week, for at least three weeks, it is likely to be colic. Unfortunately, because there are several probable causes of colic, a trial and error approach is used to treat it. Therefore consult with your health visitor after keeping a cry diary for about three weeks, but be patient as you try different remedies to see what works. Each remedy that your health visitor recommends should be tried for a week. In the meantime, try to reassure your baby as he cries and endeavour to contain his emotions. Let him know that you feel his pain and are trying to provide a solution. It is comforting to also know that colic often resolves by 3–6 months of age.

Your baby's excessive crying can be very hard for you as a parent. It is important to mention that long periods of crying may also be an indication of pain or illness. Therefore, seek medical help if this happens. If you feel that you are unable to cope with your baby's crying, try to get yourself a break and enlist the support of your family, friends or trusted neighbours. Take some time out and talk to someone you trust about how you are feeling. Speak with your health visitor who can also provide support. You don't have to struggle alone.

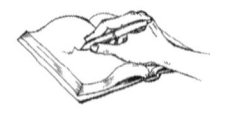

Please turn to the Appendix and look for the heading *Could It be Colic?*

> *'Trust yourself. You know more than you think you do.'*
> Benjamin Spock, Paediatrician

Sleeping

All humans, adults and children alike sleep in cycles ranging from drowsiness to light sleep, then deep sleep followed by

TUNE IN TO YOUR BABY

dream sleep (REM - Rapid Eye Movement). Between light sleep and deep sleep is a stage called quiet sleep (Non Rapid Eye Movement), during which we may dream. Over the total period of a night a person may have five sleep cycles. A newborn's sleep cycle is between 50-60 minutes long. By three months of age, this will increase to 90-minute cycles, the same as an adult.

Between each sleep cycle there is a brief awakening which is essential for our survival. If when we wake up everything is as we expect it to be and there is no change in our environment since we fell asleep, we will quickly fall back to sleep and have no recollection of waking up. The same applies to your baby. Sometimes, your baby may wake up between cycles and not go back to sleep, because their surroundings have changed. For example your child may have fallen asleep in your arms and awakens between sleep cycles to find himself in his cot and you are not there. He may become upset to find this change, and will cry or call out for you to return. This is called a sleep association. Sleep associations, like rocking baby to sleep or baby falling asleep on the breast are difficult to break once they've become a habit. It is thus best to teach your baby to sleep by himself. It is important to have a good bedtime routine as it will teach your baby that it's time to wind down. This should last only about 20–30 minutes in order not to stimulate your baby.

Once baby is ready for bed, settle your baby down to sleep without talking to them too much. If he wants a drink, offer water, but not milk. Leave him in his cot, bid them good night and walk away. Your baby may cry. This is alright. He misses you and wants you to know. But he will eventually learn to self-soothe and go to sleep on his own. Let him cry for about five minutes before checking on him. Gradually increase the time your baby is left before checking. If you persist in the routine, your baby should learn to fall asleep by himself in no time. If however, you do not persist, it will take longer to teach your baby to learn to sleep on his own. This is where delayed gratification can help you. Whilst it is painful watching your child cry, by focusing on the long-term gains, you can enable him to develop good sleep habits.

You are Your Baby's Teacher!

One of the roles you have as a parent is to teach your child new skills. In the first few years of life you will teach your child everything your baby needs to learn for survival - how to eat, sleep, walk, talk, etc. Children often learn by copying their parents' example. Therefore, it is important to model good behaviour. If you want your child to learn to eat healthily, you should do the same. If you want your child to drink water, you should drink water. If you want your child to develop healthy sleep habits, you should do the same. Even if you get away with not setting a good example, before long your child will get wiser and eventually start to copy your example. Once bad habits are formed, they take longer to unlearn.

As has already been established, it is not easy to teach your baby a new skill. The key to ensuring your baby learns what you want to teach them is consistency and persistence. For example if you want to teach your baby to sleep by himself, you have to perform the same bedtime routine every night. If you keep changing your baby's routine, this can give your baby mixed messages and cause confusion for him, thus, the need for consistency. Secondly, because habits are hard to change, you need to be persistent. Your baby was previously used to sleeping in your room and had developed a habit of sleeping close to you. Moving him into his own room is a new habit you want him to develop, but one that he is not used to. By being persistent, he will learn that this is the new routine or habit and he will eventually adapt to it. However, this is easier said than done, as it can be an emotional time for both you and your little one. By staying committed to enjoying the parenting experience, you will be able to take the good sides of parenting and the challenging aspects such as watching your baby cry. By being firm but positive, your baby will learn to trust you and eventually work with you.

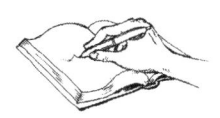

Please turn to the appendix and look for the heading *Teaching My Baby.*

Get Organised!

Manage Your Time

As a parent, you may sometimes wish you have more than 24 hours in a day. Before the birth of your baby you had 24 hours each day to lead a busy life. Now that your baby is here you still have the same amount of time but much more to do. Caring for your baby is taking so much of your time, that it leaves you tired with very little time for yourself. If you are feeling this way, it may be worthwhile to review how you spend your time. Like money, you can't spend time that you don't have. However, when it comes to time there are no credit cards that you can borrow and pay off later. What tends to happen is that you eat into time that you should spend on essential things like sleep. While this may be all right for a few days, if this continues over time, you will begin to suffer from sleep deprivation. Whilst we may underestimate the effects of sleep deprivation, there is a very good reason that it is often used as a form of torture: it works! One of the symptoms of prolonged sleep deprivation is hallucinations. Sleep is needed to regenerate certain parts of the body, especially the brain, for optimum functioning. Neurons (nerve cells) may begin to malfunction, after periods of extended wakefulness or reduced sleep, visibly affecting a person's behaviour (Serendip, 2008).

As sleep occurs in cycles, it is important to get enough hours of sleep in order to get deep, restorative sleep. Without restorative sleep, you will become like a car that is overheating. If you fail to allow the car to cool down, the engine can pack up. Rest is also important because some parts of the body like muscles are able to regenerate even when a person is not sleeping, as long as they are resting. Sleep debt (the difference between the amount of sleep you need and the hours you actually sleep), like any other debt will need to be repaid. Eventually the sleep 'account' has to balance. So how can you manage your time so that you do not dip into time required for essential things?

Pareto Principle (The 80:20 Rule)

The well-known Pareto principle (also known as the 80:20 rule) is a powerful idea that is universally applicable in practically every sphere of our lives. It implies that 20 per cent of your effort will generate 80 per cent of your results and that the remaining 80 per cent of effort generates the last 20 per cent of results. Consequently, only 20 per cent of the things you do are vital or essential for achieving results, the other 80 per cent are trivial or non-essential. The key is to identify and focus on the 20 per cent that matters, as they produce 80 per cent of your results. So establish your 20 per cent and give them your top priority, then concentrate on them.

I'll quickly illustrate this. It's essential to eat, sleep, care for your baby, and exercise. When you ensure that these things are included in your daily 20 per cent you will find that you perform better as a parent. If you replace one of the essential things such as sleeping with a non-essential thing like watching television, you sleep less and will eventually get tired which may affect your ability to care for your little one. I did not realise how important this principle was until I tried it. I found myself getting exhausted but it was not due to sleep as I love my sleep, but to a lack of exercise. I became sluggish and not as sharp as I'd like to be. I incorporated just 30 minutes of exercise into my daily routine and the results were astounding. Within a month I had more energy and was able to do more. I slept better and woke up in the morning with a spring in my step. My moods were better and I was able to parent better as I was less irritable and more tolerant of my son's tantrums. So I implore you to try it. You may be surprised how much difference it can make to your life as a parent.

Determine your 20 per cent and do it!

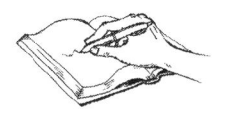

Please turn to the appendix and look for the heading – *'Find Your 20 Per Cent!'*

Plan Your Day, Daily!

It is important to plan each day as it allows you to include time for essential people and things. It also allows you to create a clear path for yourself that maintains a healthy balance of work and play. Planning your day can reduce stress and increase peace of mind. It also helps you prepare for hurdles as you often have to create a contingency plan for unexpected problems. Further, it helps you to evaluate your progress as you go through the day and gives you a feeling of fulfilment as you check things off. When you plan, see your day going the best way possible. It gives you the right mindset to tackle it.

When you plan, incorporate your baby's routines into your day. Over time both you and baby will get used to the routine. This will create safety and stability for your baby as he will know what to expect.

It is also a good habit to review how your day has gone. Over the course of the day you may find that you have some successes and some things that did not go so well. By reflecting at the end of the day, you will discover what you've succeeded at, learned and what you will change. I call this *Successes, Learns and Changes (SLC)*. I keep a daily journal about this and at the end of each day, I review and fix it. Then I plan the next day just before I go to bed. I see my next day going the best way possible and then I go to sleep. When I awake I find that I feel very positive. Over the course of a few months, I look back and discover how much I've grown and it is exciting. Whilst there is no guarantee that this will work for you, it is worth a try as I find that keeping a positive mindset prepares you for the day rather than leaving it to chance.

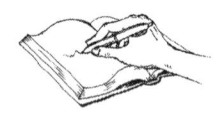

Please turn to the Appendix and look for the heading *My Daily Planner*.

Be Balanced

Parenthood often puts a strain on your relationships. This is often because raising a baby consumes a great deal of your time. It is important to remember that parenting is not your life; it is just one aspect of it. Motherhood is just one of the many roles you have. You had a life before you had a baby and you should still have one after. It is vital to manage your other roles. You are not just a mother, but probably someone's partner, daughter, sister, friend, or colleague too. Therefore ensure that you invest in your other relationships by making time for them. When you do, it is easier to call on them when you need extra support. It is often not the amount of time that matters, but the quality of time spent together. In view of this, plan to spend quality time with the significant others in your life. Take time to communicate with them regularly and remember to listen as much as you speak. Let them know how you are feeling, but be prepared to let them air their feelings too. If you have relatives, get them to babysit so that you can spend time alone with your partner. Doing things together can strengthen your bond. Also ensure that your partner gets to spend time alone with your baby. Not only does it give you some time for you, but it also gives your partner the opportunity to parent your child and you the chance to show that you trust your partner is able to care for him. When a load is shared, it becomes easier to bear. Share parenting your infant with those that matter to you as long as they do not take over and try to undermine your role as a parent.

It is often said that 'you lose some, you gain some'. The same is true for motherhood. Motherhood is a time when you may lose friends especially if they are not mothers too. Remember that it is not the number of friends you have, but the quality of the friendships. You may also gain friendships as you may meet other mothers at postnatal groups, mum and toddler groups, playgroups or nursery.

> *'It's not what you are that holds you back, it's what you think you are not'*
>
> Denis Waitley, Motivational speaker and writer

Trust That Things Will Eventually Fall Into Place

I recently listened to a Stanford Commencement Speech, made by Steve Jobs, and it really resonated with me as a parent. In it he stated,

'Trust that the dots will connect. You can't connect the dots looking forward. You can only connect them looking backwards, so you have to trust that the dots will somehow connect in your future. You have to trust in something – gut instinct, whatever – because believing that the dots will connect down the road will give you the confidence to follow your heart, even when it leads you off the well-worn path, and that will make all the difference'.

When you first hold your child, you get a scary feeling when you consider the huge responsibility that comes with having a baby. You get anxious. Everyone tells you that you will be fine. But somehow you don't believe it. Over time as you grow into your role you look back and wonder what the worry was all about but that does not stop you from worrying when you are faced with the next challenge as a parent. My advice to you is that you should trust your instincts, as it will all fall into place. In the meantime, celebrate every day that you succeed as a parent. There will be challenges but trust that you will handle them. As you cope with them, you will develop your parenting muscles and grow in confidence. Every day, focus on your strengths and not your problems, stay positive and enjoy your role as a parent of your baby.

When Things Don't Go to Plan

As in pregnancy, not everything goes to plan after you have had your baby. Although there are many things that may not go as expected, I will focus on only four of these and suggests some strategies that can help you to cope if you find yourself in any of these situations. It is important that you deal with these problems quickly as not doing so can prevent you from tuning in to your baby.

If you experience any negative feelings that you are concerned about, then please read the section entitled Important Notice.

Loneliness

You may feel cut off from your old friends and have difficulty making new ones. You may have family but they are not close by. Your partner may have gone back to work. All of a sudden you feel isolated, despite having your baby as a companion. Again, it is important to remember that you are not alone. Many mothers feel lonely especially after the birth of their first child. A reason for this is that we tend to focus more on our pregnancy than we do on becoming a mum, so we may not be prepared when our baby actually arrives. How then can you deal with loneliness after the birth of your baby? As you are not alone, try to find other mums just like you. Being able to share the ups and downs of motherhood with others in the *same shoes* as you can help you cope. Speak to your health visitor and ask for information about local groups for mothers and babies. Whilst waiting to be seen at child health clinics, chat with the other mums that you see. There are also many online parenting forums that you can access. Contact your health visitor for a list of these.

Postnatal Depression

Postnatal depression is not to be confused with the *baby blues* which many women get after their baby is born. Baby blues normally occur in the first few days after the birth of your baby. It is caused by the sudden hormonal and chemical change that takes place after birth. Symptoms include feeling irritable, weepy for no reason, anxious, low in mood, emotional and irrational. This is normal and lasts only a few days.

Unlike the baby blues, postnatal depression does not just go away. It usually occurs between 2–8 weeks after birth but can start anytime up to a year after the birth of your baby. Symptoms may include anxiety, depression, panic attacks, sleeplessness, forgetfulness, lack of concentration, feeling like you can't cope, constant crying, losing interest in things, yourself and baby, feelings of hopelessness, loss of appetite and undue anxiety about your baby.

Postnatal depression affects one in every 7 to 10 mothers. Although the exact cause of postnatal depression is unknown, it is more common in mothers who have previously had episodes of depression or have a family history of depression. It is also more common in mothers who have experienced stressful life events during the pregnancy, mothers who feel unsupported, in those in whom the baby was unplanned or unwanted, and when the baby has been born with some problem.

Despite the above, postnatal depression can be treated. If you have it, there is no need to struggle alone. It is not a reflection of your parenting. It is an illness like any other, so ask for help. See your doctor or health visitor. It is easier to treat postnatal depression early before it spirals out of control. Therefore seek early help and accept it when it is offered. Enlist the help of your partner and family. Maintain a healthy diet and ensure you get enough sleep and rest. In severe cases, postnatal depression may require treatment with anti-depressants. If you are breast-feeding, inform your doctor about this. Remember that it is not your fault that you are ill and with the right support and treatment you will soon put the illness behind you.

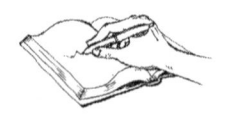

Please turn to the Appendix and look for the heading *Managing My Feelings*.

> *'Do you want to be right, or do you want to be happy? Forgive yourself and stop punishing yourself.'*
>
> Louise L. Hay, Author and publisher

Domestic Abuse

One in four women experience domestic abuse at some point in their lives (Council of Europe, 2002). Although men can be victims of domestic abuse, research shows that women are most often the victims. Any woman can experience domestic abuse regardless of race, ethnic or religious group, class, disability or lifestyle. It can take the form of physical, sexual, psychological, emotional or financial abuse. It often takes place within an intimate or family type relationship and stems from the abuser's desire for power and control over you. Signs of domestic abuse include verbal abuse, disrespect, pressure tactics, breaking trust, isolation, harassment, threats, physical or sexual violence or denial. Nearly a third of domestic abuse begins in pregnancy, and existing abuse may worsen in pregnancy or after baby's birth. It puts a woman's health and that of her baby at risk. Therefore, no one should have to put up with it. When children witness domestic abuse, it can have a detrimental effect on them.

If you experience domestic abuse you don't need to suffer alone as help and support are readily available. You are not to blame for the abuse. Speak with your midwife, doctor or health visitor who can assist in protecting you and your children and enable you to feel safe. There are local support services and a confidential 24-hour National Domestic Abuse helpline that can provide you with information and support.

RUTH OSHIKANLU

> *'Never begin the day until it is finished on paper'*
>
> Jim Rohn, Entrepreneur, author and motivational speaker

Relationship Breakdown – Single Parenting

You read Chapter 1 and were probably wondering what happened to me and Joshua's dad. Well, the difficult pregnancy put a strain on our relationship. Despite his support in pregnancy and after Joshua was born, our relationship broke down. I didn't realise how much my difficult pregnancy and long hospitalisation had affected him. Whilst I was worrying about myself and my unborn baby, and being stuck on a hospital bed, he had to worry about all that plus keep a full-time job whilst catering for my needs. After Joshua was born we tried to resolve our issues and make our relationship work, but soon came to realise that we were in it for the wrong reasons. It was sad for both of us but we tried to keep our baby in mind. Our main priority was Joshua's happiness and wellbeing and we did not want to damage him in any way by staying together. Even though it was a joint decision it was not easy. The feelings of 'I didn't plan for this' came back and it was not easy to bear. Having been raised by two parents, a part of me felt a failure. I was now faced with the task of raising Joshua alone.

Even though I am a lone parent, I must say that I have never felt alone. My parents and brothers have been a source of immense support. Joshua's dad has also been supportive and Joshua spends time with him every other weekend. I have also built up a support network of very close friends, many of whom are themselves, single parents.

If you find yourself in a similar situation, you do not have to be alone. If you have family and friends living close by, ask them for help. Seek the support of other single parents and your ex-partner. There are also many lone parent support organisations that can assist you to manage as a single parent. Rather than focusing on what you don't have such as companionship and a shared responsibility, focus on the benefits of being a lone parent. As a single parent you have greater control over what you decide for your family and do not have the conflict that two parent families may experience when there are differing views on parenting. Having total financial control can be a huge relief if you were with a partner that was financially irresponsible. A single mum is often able to focus on her children's best interests without distractions or conflicting opinions from a partner getting in the way. Single parents often have more independence and freedom. Their children also learn increased independence as because there is only one parent, they often have to learn to do things by themselves at an earlier age than children of two-parent families. Spending time in two different home environments will also teach the child to be flexible, resilient and adaptable; skills which will benefit them later in life. So single parenting isn't all bad! Make it what you want it to be.

Don't Become a Victim

When things do not go as planned as a parent, it is often easy to say poor me and wallow in self-pity. We refuse to take responsibility for ourselves and unconsciously choose to react as a victim. This inevitably creates feelings of anger, fear, guilt or inadequacy and leaves us feeling betrayed, or taken advantage of by others. In the drama triangle, Karpman described three roles on an inverted triangle – Persecutor, Rescuer and Victim. Persecutors and Rescuers act from a one-up position. Persecutors put people down, whilst Rescuers discount a person's ability to be able to work things out for themselves. Victims act from a one-down position and discount their own ability to do things or work things out for themselves. They believe themselves to be victims of other people.

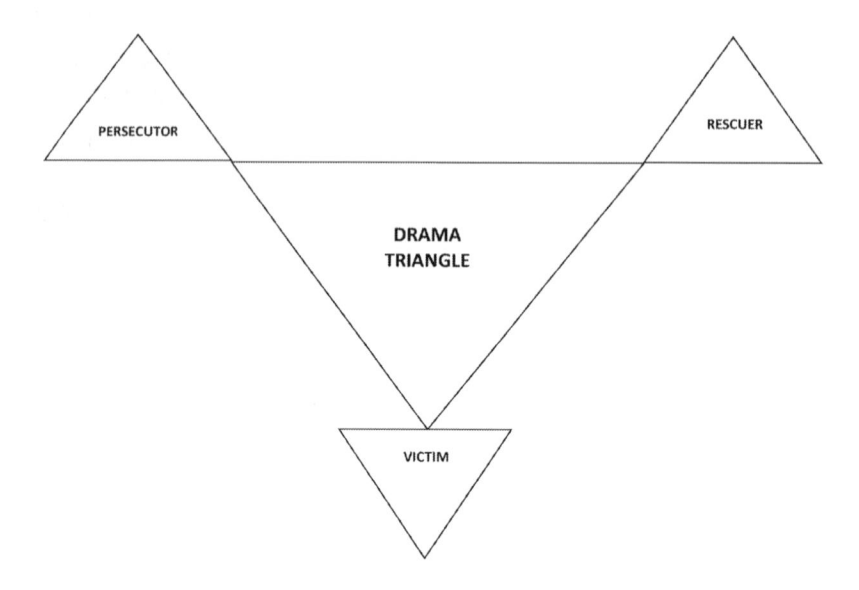

```
         PERSECUTOR                          RESCUER

                     DRAMA
                   TRIANGLE

                     VICTIM
```

The Drama Triangle

According to Michael Bradford, victims often believe that they have no power and that nothing positive will ever happen for them. Their focus is on the past and negativity. They spend endless hours talking about their problems, and how things are never right and there is never enough. They feel helpless, hopeless, and tend to be confused, living in constant fear of making a mistake or looking foolish. They always have an excuse for not doing things.

If you find yourself acting in this way, it may be difficult to break the cycle. Habits such as thinking negatively can be difficult to break. If we continually think in a particularly way, it becomes a pattern – a thinking pattern. Notwithstanding this, you have the power to change habits that are not serving you with those that do. You can develop wholesome ways of thinking when you are ready to take full responsibility for all of your thoughts. This will in turn influence your feelings, and actions. Make an effort to improve your attitude towards change, control, and responsibility. Instead of looking to others for approval or what is right, look inward. Endeavour to become genuine and true to yourself. Don't let others set yours standards. Welcome change and see life as a learning experience. Remain open and curious. Allow yourself to make mistakes and learn from them. Give yourself the permission to feel out of control as you will grow as you find your own solutions.

Please turn to the appendix and look for the heading *Breaking My Thinking Pattern*.

Not Yet! No Such Thing as Failure!

OK. so things didn't go to plan. You don't have to stay the course of the plan. Plans have natural lives. If you find that your plan is not working, it is probably because it has run its course, and is now outdated. Therefore, you need to change plan. Make another one. In this way, none of your plans will fail but just evolve into other plans. So for instance, you are trying to lose some pregnancy weight and get back in shape. You have made a plan to lose weight. Initially you lose some weight. But after a while, you stop losing weight without getting to your target weight. Has your plan failed? No! You make another plan or keep adjusting the old plan until you get the desired outcome. You may not have got to your desired weight yet, but you will if you persist.

Your baby will often use this approach when learning new skills, such as learning to walk. Baby falls, baby gets up. Over and over again, baby falls and gets up until he learns how to stand and eventually walk. Not once during this process does your baby fall and stay on the floor, viewing himself as a failure and refusing to try again. So why should you? If things don't go according to your initial plan, adapt it and keep trying until you get to where you want to be.

Going Back to Work

Your maternity leave is over and the time has come for you to go back to work. This can be another time of great anxiety. Not only do you have to face the fear of the unknown, there is the doubt about whether you will ever be able to cope at work - the emotional upheaval of leaving your baby, the adjustment to your new role as mother, the organisation required to get to work on time and collect your child at the end of the day, the worry whether your baby will be alright without you and the guilt about leaving your child with someone else.

I returned to work when my son was almost a year old to train as a health visitor. In order to ensure that my son was adequately cared for, I must have checked out about 20 nurseries. I loved the first nursery that I saw as it was a small one that employed a home from home approach. Despite this, I felt the need to view another 19 or so. I had acquired a list of all the registered childcare providers in the borough and felt obligated to view as many as possible. In order to ensure that I was not leaving my baby with strangers by the time I was ready to go back to work, Joshua started nursery part-time for two days a week when he was seven months. I recall the first day I had to leave him by himself. I must have called the nursery every hour to check up on him. Eventually, Joshua settled into the nursery within three weeks. Despite this, the day before returning to work I felt a great deal of anxiety and spent the whole day entertaining doubts about my decision to return to work. A great lack of confidence overcame me as I felt that I would no longer be competent at work due to the long period of not working – almost 18 months. I had never been out of work for this length of time, hence, the apprehension.

The week before, I planned my route to work to ensure that I would be able to make it to work on time and get back to pick Joshua up afterwards. Despite all my preparation, there was one thing I didn't prepare for – the guilt!

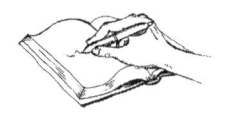

Please turn to the appendix and look for the heading I'm Going Back to Work – Plan For Success!

Guilt – Use It or Lose It!

Joshua had been at nursery for two days a week for about three months when I returned to work. I didn't feel guilty because I felt that I was still caring for him most of the time. The first day I left him, knowing that he was going to be cared for by the nursery full-time because I was returning to work made me feel incredibly guilty. I cried as I left him, as I kept thinking there must be another way. I kept asking whether I really needed or even wanted to be a health visitor. In the first week of the year-long programme, the university lecturers kept stressing how hard the course would be and how committed we had to be to complete the programme. I'm sure they said other things, but that's the main thing I heard. I still had doubts whether I had done the right thing. Because I felt guilty, even though I wanted to stop breast-feeding, I continued probably due to guilt. I felt that as I could not care for him during the day, by breast-feeding him, I would make up for it. Over the time the guilt improved as Joshua and I settled into our new routines. On reflection, I ask myself why the guilt?

Guilt appears to be an inherent part of parenting. We feel guilty about doing things to our children, such as disciplining, or not doing things for our children such as not spending as much time as we would love to spend with them. Guilt in itself is not a bad thing as it can be a warning sign that you have to change direction. It can be a useful teacher, letting you know that you need to step back and look at the whole picture. For example, after qualifying as a health visitor, I got a job that involved me working long hours. It was a role that involved enabling young mothers to parent their young babies. In the morning I would leave my young toddler sleeping. In the evening, I would leave work feeling really good about the difference I was making to the lives of my clients only to get home when my son was asleep in bed. I would feel an incredible sense of guilt telling myself that I was busy helping others to parent when I couldn't even parent mine. Over time the feelings of guilt worsened. Even though I loved the job so much, it had to go as it was preventing me from parenting my son to the best of my ability. So the guilt served a purpose. It made me improve my perspective and change course. When guilt is used in this way, it is healthy.

However, there are times when guilt can be incapacitating. Some parents feel guilty about everything that goes wrong for their children. They feel they are not good enough and want to be perfect. They worry about all the things that they could have done better and find evidence to confirm it. So they've gone back to work leaving their child with the child-minder and missed their child's first step. They feel guilty. They must be bad parents for leaving their child in the care of someone else. So their *'punishment'* is that they miss out on witnessing their child's development milestones. This is when I feel guilt becomes unhealthy. Guilt can be likened to a parasitic plant.

Once it begins climbing up a tree, its roots and suckers dig in tightly absorbing all the nutrients and clinging tightly to the host plant. It's hard to let go of guilt, because guilt won't let go of you. At this point guilt is not serving you. It is not helping you move forward, but causing you to get stuck and gradually to eat away at you. This is where I suggest that you have to lose it! When you feel guilty, ask yourself if you can change the situation. If you can, then do. If not, lose the guilt! Don't let guilt rob you of the joys of parenting.

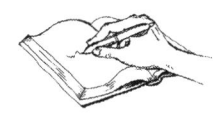

Please turn to the appendix and look for the heading *Why the Guilt?*

> 'If you can control your behaviour when everything around you is out of control, you can model for your children a valuable lesson in patience and understanding ... and snatch an opportunity to shape character.'
>
> Jane Clayson Johnson, Journalist and author

Work/Life Balance

When you return to work after the birth of your baby, it is important that you balance your role as a parent and as a worker. Otherwise, one may impact on the other. How can you do this? It is important to plan and prepare for your return to work. Anything that causes you to feel guilty about leaving your child in the care of someone else may impact on your performance at work. Ensure that you have good childcare arrangements and a backup plan for childcare in case of emergencies. If you are still breast-feeding your child, you can continue with good planning and the support of your employer and childcare providers. It is important to make time for your child. Even the best childcare is not a substitute for parenting. Spend quality time with your child as often as you can. Incorporate it into your routine and your child will come to expect it. Do things together as often as you can.

As a working parent you will have two full-time jobs. You'll finish your paid job and then get home and start your unpaid job as a parent. We sometimes forget that some of the skills we utilise in our day jobs are transferable to our lives at home. We may communicate well at work but somehow not so well at home. We may manage our time at work, but not so well at home. So look for the skills that you use at work and transfer them to use at home and vice versa.

In order not to burn out, set your priorities. Decide what is important and focus on these. Neglecting important things will make those things urgent later. It is important to communicate with your partner, if you have one. You know what you are thinking and how you are feeling, so don't bottle it up. Try to share things like the housework and childcare if possible. Get the support of your employer and familiarise yourself with your employer's work policies. Take advantage of family-friendly working arrangements if they offer them. Endeavour to enjoy your life at home and at work. Remember to look after yourself as there is only one of you.

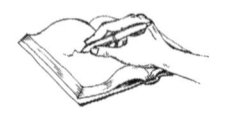

Please turn to the appendix and look for the heading *Home and Work Swap*.

Continue Loving, Playing and Learning with Your Baby

Playtime is a time for you as a parent to relax and unwind. It is fun and helps you to focus on what is truly important: your child. Play helps you better understand what your child likes and his abilities. When playing with your child, give your child your undivided attention. Immerse yourself in the activity, allow your child to take the lead and enjoy being a kid again. Allow your child to choose the play activity and take the lead. He is more likely to maintain interest for longer. Remember that your child has a short attention span.

Play also helps your baby develop his confidence. Incorporate play into your baby's daily routine, such as bath time, mealtimes, cooking, etc. Endeavour to make every activity fun. As children learn through play, encourage your child to learn by encouraging new challenges. When playing with a new toy, resist the urge to help him. Let him try first. If he continues to struggle, show him how it's done, but then give it back to him so he can try again on his own. When he succeeds, give him lots of praise.

Let your baby know how much you love him. Shower him with love and affection. Smiles, kisses, hugs and cuddles are ways you can demonstrate love to your baby. Reaffirm it by telling him you love him, stating the reasons why you do. If you started in pregnancy, continue talking to your child. If not, start now. Research shows that children whose parents spoke to them extensively as babies have significantly higher IQs and richer vocabularies than those who didn't receive much verbal stimulation. Therefore, talk about anything and everything with your child and observe his reaction. According to Albert Mehrabian, when we talk, the meaning of a message is communicated by our words (7%), our tone of voice (38%) and our body language (55%). Thus your baby does not require words to communicate. Observe his body language when you speak and you will be able to pick up his response. In order for your child to learn the art of conversation and taking turns to speak, always pause for a response from your child. Before long when you pause he will start cooing or babbling.

Read aloud to your baby. It helps promote your child's speech and helps build his vocabulary, stimulate his imagination, and improve his language skills. However, be careful not to overstimulate your little one. Look out for any cues that may show that your baby wants to disengage and stop the activity. The more you develop the habit of reading to your baby, the more you will instil a love of books and learning in him.

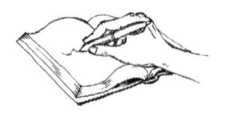

Please turn to the appendix and look for the heading *More Loving, Playing and Learning.*

Raising a baby is not easy but be determined to enjoy parenting yours. When you do it will be easier to tune in to him.

Sharing My Learning

- Perfect parenting is an illusion. It doesn't exist. Accept it, so that you don't set yourself up to fail.
- Embrace being a good *enough* parent.
- Learn from your mistakes – we often first learn how not to do things before we learn how to do them.
- Your baby is unique, so don't compare!
- Make adult decisions.
- Be patient and view each day as a learning experience.
- Delayed gratification pays more than instant gratification.
- Trust that things will eventually fall into place.
- Get organised and manage your time.
- Remember that 20 per cent of what you do creates 80 per cent of your results. Determine your 20 per cent and do it!
- Plan your day on a daily basis.
- Be balanced and manage all your relationships.
- You are your baby's teacher, so model good behaviour.
- Be consistent and persistent.
- Be committed to enjoying the parenting experience.
- When things don't go to plan, don't become a victim, make another plan. Keep trying until you succeed and ask for help if you need it. Often, those you need help from are only a telephone call away.

- Going back to work can make you feel guilty so learn to manage it. Plan for it and ensure you maintain your work/life balance.
- Continue to love, play and learn with your baby.

> *'When you make a mistake, don't look back at it for long. Take the reason of the thing into your mind, and then look forward. Mistakes are lessons of wisdom. The past cannot be changed. The future is yet in your power.'*
>
> Hugh White, Politician

Chapter 5

Help, My Child Has Mutated! The Toddler Years

This is what I said when Joshua changed from being a contented, compliant little baby to a toddler that wanted to do everything I didn't want him to and wouldn't do anything I wanted him to. It was a very challenging time as I was so unprepared for it. It appeared to have happened almost overnight. One day my Joshua was predictable, the next day he was not. I had heard about the terrible twos but Joshua did not wait until two before he started exhibiting toddler behaviour. He started at about 15 months. This was the first time since his birth that I experienced any difficulty parenting Joshua because of his behaviour. Before now, the problems were on my part, my anxieties and insecurities as a parent, not being sure what to do. But this time, it felt like a battle and somehow I took it personally. Joshua appeared to be on a mission to make my life difficult. It also didn't help that I was halfway through my health visitor training and as such was busy with my studies.

You, too, might find the toddler years challenging as your toddler may start to refuse food, become fussy in eating, start having tantrums, not want to sleep or start waking in the night after previously sleeping through. Thus, in this chapter I will discuss why a toddler behaves the way he does so that once again you can tune in to him to find what his needs are. I will also consider some of the challenging behaviours that a toddler may exhibit and suggest some strategies to help you to manage them. I will start with defining what toddlerhood is in order to prepare you for this time.

What are the Toddler Years?

Although toddlerhood is referred to as the terrible twos it often starts before then. A toddler is a little person aged between one and four years. By one year of age many children are walking with or without support and are ready to explore their environment. They can also feed themselves with finger foods and by 13 months they are ready to feed themselves very messily with a spoon. At the same time they are able to take off easily removable clothes like socks, hats and gloves. Because toddlers are very inquisitive, they are impulsive and do not give thought to their actions. When your child was a baby, he spent a long time observing what you did, but was unable to copy all that you did as he had limited ability and mobility. Now your toddler is able to do more and can also move about, his newfound freedom enables him to copy more of what you do. He thinks to himself, if you can do it, why can't I? When you object, he tries to exert his authority, almost as if to say who are you to tell me what to do? This can make it really challenging for you as a parent especially as this behaviour happens suddenly. The problem is that toddlers have lots of energy and need to expend it. Yet they have little sense. They do not understand risk or danger, but want to explore their surroundings. Thus, it is vital for parents to ensure that they enable their toddlers to develop by making sure that their environment is safe for them to do so. As a toddler develops, he also develops his speech and can now talk back. By the time he is two years old, he may understand up to fifty words and can often put two words together. He knows much more than he knew before and thinks he now knows it all. As a result he wants independence.

Going back to Maslow's hierarchy of needs, which we considered in Chapter 2, your toddler has reached the peak of the triangle and thinks he has self-actualised and wants independence from you. Since his conception he has been dependent on you. He was born and was then still reliant on you first for survival and then for love. As you proved yourself as a parent, he started to trust you. You continuously told him how much you loved him, but didn't stop at that. You proved you loved him by your actions. He now knows you love him so dearly and he trusts and loves you, but he feels the need to find himself and be free from you. He has the ability to move around. He is curious and wants to explore his surroundings. He has kept all your rules before now because he felt he didn't have a choice: he needed you. Now he feels he does not need you. All he wants is to be the centre of attention. He knows that since his birth your world has revolved around him. He loves that and wants that to continue. If he could have your attention 110 per cent at all times he would love that. The difference now is that he wants to do things his way and not just yours. As a result, he doesn't care how he makes you feel as long as he gets his way. What matters to him is that his needs are met and that he is happy, regardless of how you feel. Besides, a toddler has a short attention span and lives only for the moment. He does not think about the consequences of his actions. What he cares for is to satisfy his curiosity regardless of the outcome.

Due to your toddler's need for independence, you may now find that he has problems eating, sleeping and may start to have tantrums. This can be quite distressing for you as a parent especially if you have gone back to work, are a lone parent or both. Thus, the next section will discuss why fussy eating, sleeping problems and tantrums happen and how you can manage them.

Fussy Eating – Why it Happens

Toddlers need a varied, balanced diet to grow and develop properly. From about 12 months, feeding a toddler can become more difficult as this is when the neophobic (fear of new) stage starts. At this stage, a toddler rejects new foods or previously accepted food on sight. Before the toddler can eat food, it has to pass the sight test. The food doesn't look good and so he rejects it. It may just be due to presentation. The child may have tried and liked the food before, but now it looks different, so he won't try it as it doesn't look safe. I remember on one occasion, Joshua saying that the food was dirty when he saw some thyme on the rice I had cooked him. He kept refusing to eat the food even though he liked to eat rice, but the little specks of herb that were on the food had contaminated it making it unsafe. Even after picking them out he wouldn't eat it as in his eyes, the food was polluted, firstly with the thyme and secondly with my hands.

> *'Live for the present, dream of the future, learn from the past.'*
> Unknown

How to Manage Fussy Eating

The good news is that this stage does not last. The neophobia (fear of new) stage decreases with age; by the time your child is five years old, he should have very few neophobic responses. Unfortunately, though, the number of exposures required to induce a food preference increases with age. With a baby, you will only have to offer a new food once or twice for him to acquire a taste for it. Whereas with a toddler, you may have to try a new food about 14 times or more, before he acquires a taste for it. A great deal of patience and persistence is thus required from you as the parent. Another way that you can encourage your child to eat new foods is for him to see you eating them. Toddlers can often tell if a parent is being hypocritical with food and will often tell their parents to eat the food first. So if you want your child to eat broccoli that is good for them, you have to eat it too. And you can see the reason why. If broccoli is good for your child, it's good for you too! So when it comes to eating, be a good role model. When your child also mixes with other children such as older siblings or other children at nursery and sees them eating healthy foods, they are more likely to imitate them.

The way a parent manages mealtimes is also important. According to Gillian Harris, parents often tend to adopt three main feeding styles when it comes to mealtime management.

Authoritarian parents adopt a 'do as I say' approach. They will force the child to sit and eat what is in front of them, giving the child no choice. The child wants his independence and protests against this and mealtimes are not a pleasurable experience. The parents use more force and overpower the toddler who eventually unhappily succumbs.

Permissive parents are the complete opposite and do not challenge the toddler, letting him have his own way. They do not introduce new tastes and textures to the toddler and, as I discussed in the previous chapter, this has its limitations. It makes introducing new foods later on more challenging as the child has now become used to always having his way.

Sitting between the two is the **authoritative** parent who makes confident suggestions for their toddler. They don't use force, neither do they allow the toddler to have his own way. They are firm and loving. The child recognises this and works with them. This is the style that it is best to adopt when it comes to feeding your toddler. If your child does not eat, do not make a fuss. It's probably because he is not hungry. When children are well, they will usually eat when they are hungry. So take the food away without making a fuss and offer it again later. If your toddler realises that mealtimes are difficult for you to manage, he will use this against you. Remember, that your child wants your attention. He doesn't care how he gets it. If he knows winding you up will get him some attention, he will do so.

It is also important to stress portion sizes. Over the years we as adults now eat more and our plate sizes have grown with our increased appetite. Sometimes, parents complain that their toddlers do not eat enough, but this is because their parents want them to eat more food than they need. In reality a portion of food is roughly how much can fit in the palms of our hands. But we eat much more than that and expect our toddlers to do the same. When they don't, we as parents, worry about it. Therefore, as a rough guide, if your child is eating portion sizes that are about the size of his little palm, he his eating enough for his little stomach. Don't put him off his food by the amount of food you offer him!

Finally, I want to discuss the habit of using food as a reward. Often in exasperation, parents resort to bribing their children with food. I did this too, before I realised how unproductive it was and even worse, the use of food as a comforter. I remember bribing Joshua that if he ate all of his vegetables, I would give him pudding. Remember, that your toddler wants to do the opposite of what you want him to do. So when you restrict a preferred food, you actually increase your toddler's preference for it, it becomes more desirable. So you tell your child that he will not have his pudding until he has all his vegetables, now all he wants is the pudding. Rather than use food as a reward, assign a specific time of the day when you will offer such treats so that your toddler will not associate it with anything in particular. Most importantly, make mealtimes fun and eat together as a family. Your child will learn from you – not just what to eat but how to eat – good table manners. As your child grows older, make the food you will eat together. Making a face out of fruits and challenge your toddler to eat the face starting with the eyes. He will see it more as a game, and before he knows it he has eaten a little plate of fruit effortlessly.

If your toddler continues to have problems with eating after trying the above suggestions, speak with your health visitor who can provide you with extra support. One thing the health visitor will want to do is establish what your toddler's pattern of eating is. She may ask you to complete a food diary.

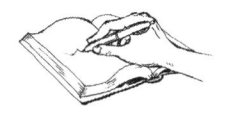

Please turn to the appendix and look for the heading *My Toddler's Food Diary*.

Sleeping Problems – Why They Happen

It can be very exhausting for a parent when a child does not sleep and hence the parent doesn't either. Although there are different types of sleep problems, I will focus on only three, mainly because these are the problems common to parents from my experience as a health visitor. These are: when your child won't settle to sleep after you have put him to bed; your toddler keeps waking up in the middle of the night; and your child keeps crawling into your bed in the middle of the night.

As was already stated in the previous chapter, your child loves you and if he had his way, he would always be with you. The feeling he experiences when he is not able to be with you is called separation anxiety and this often starts at about six to seven months and peaks between 10 and 18 months. Going back to the Maslow hierarchy of needs (the third stage on the triangle), your baby has come to love you and feels a sense of belonging to you, because of your love for him. He wants to be with you all the time and feels insecure when you are separated from him. You put him to bed and he cries, he lets you know how upset he is with you; that you've 'abandoned' him to sleep by himself. He cries and cries, to induce guilt. Then you do feel guilty and you go to pick him, reassure him and he stops. You tell him how much you love him and then put him down again. He cries even more and then you go back again and reassure him. Even when you try to extend the interval between going back to his room, he cries even louder and appears to rev up the crying engine. Eventually, you give in and he's back in your bed, or you are in his room on a mattress on the floor.

Other toddlers are fine and will settle into sleep in their beds, but will awake in the night and start crying. Because it's in the middle of the night, the cry sounds much louder and you quickly run to his room to pacify him. He feels reassured and may settle back to sleep. This may not be a problem for you as a parent, but if this becomes a common recurrence, where it is happening night after night, week after week, it may deprive you of uninterrupted sleep and leave you exhausted.

Some toddlers don't cry, especially if they are mobile. In this case, the toddler believes he is truly independent. When he was a baby, he had no choice but to cry if you were separated from him. Now that he is a toddler, he does not just have to lay there when he is put in bed to sleep. He just gets himself out of his bed and comes to meet you in your bed. He wants his way and believes he can have it. He just helps himself into your bed, convinced that you love him and won't mind. Over time, if you do not show that you mind this behaviour, it will become a habit and you can very much expect this to happen every night, especially if you feel too tired to get him out of your bed and back to his bed.

I must however, stress that there are some times when your child can awake in the night because he is sick or unwell, or there has been a change in his routine, perhaps in a new house or surroundings, or any other disruption to home life. At these times, your child's sleep may be disrupted for a period and needs you to soothe and calm him until he gets well or adjusts to his new routine.

> 'We never know the love of a parent till we become parents ourselves.'
>
> Henry Ward Beecher, Clergyman and social reformer

How to Manage Sleeping Problems

The key to managing sleep problems is to be firm with your child. Use your understanding of why a toddler does what he does to your advantage. When it comes to sleep, you are not playing games with your toddler and he needs to know this. Uninterrupted deep sleep is important for both you and your toddler and he needs to learn this. Get your toddler into a good bedtime routine and be consistent with this. You may want to try the controlled crying method. This is when you let your toddler cry for some time before going in to reassure him. Then telling him you love him and then putting him gently back to sleep. If he continues to cry, keep extending the intervals between going in to reassure him. It is important that you don't sit down to comfort your child when he is crying. That is what he wants, to get your full attention. If you do, it will become a learned habit where all he has to do is cry and he will get your undivided attention. Your child needs to learn to sleep on his own, and you have to teach him so. Although it can be hard and painful for you watching your toddler cry, the longer the sleep problems persist, the harder it is to manage.

It takes a lot of discipline to get your toddler to sleep if he tries resisting your efforts. Despite getting Joshua into a good bedtime routine, he had this power to induce guilt when I said the word bedtime. He would often refer to me as being mean, stating that it was not fair for him to go to bed when I was not going to bed too. I kept reminding him that I loved him and he needed more sleep than I did if he didn't want to wake up tired in the morning. Eventually, I would put him into bed after reading a story and giving him a good night kiss. He would cry for a short while, but amazingly within 15 minutes, he would be snoring loudly, leaving me some time for myself and to unwind before going to bed. So I'll advise you to do the same. It's not easy at first, but the hard work pays off. When you put your toddler to bed, leave straight away. If he comes out, be firm and tell him to get straight back to bed and let him know that you mean it. Try not to feel guilty about being firm. It's your responsibility as a parent to ensure that he gets enough sleep. All you are doing is fulfilling this. Act in the same way every night, unless he is unwell so that your child does not get mixed messages. It is not fair for your child when you are not consistent.

If your child keeps coming to your bed in the middle of the night, you have to decide if this is a problem for you. For me, sharing a bed with Joshua was not an option. The few times he had been in my bed due to illness, helped me reaffirm this decision as he can be quite restless in his sleep, unknowingly kicking and punching me. If you don't want your toddler to share your bed with you, it is important that you prevent this habit developing or nip it in the bud early. Let your child know that you will not tolerate this behaviour. Get up and take your toddler back to his bed. If he comes back, do the same again, firmly, letting him know that his behaviour is unacceptable. The key here is to be persistent and it will eventually pay off when your toddler realises that you mean what you say.

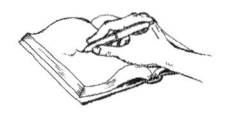

Please turn to the appendix and look for the heading *How Much Sleep Does My Toddler Get?*

Tantrums – Why They Happen

Tantrums are the hallmark of a toddler. They usually start around the time a child turns one and usually resolve by the time he is about four years of age. Tantrums range from whining and crying to screaming, throwing their toys, kicking, hitting and breath-holding, to major displays in public such as throwing themselves on the floor. Tantrums differ from child to child because each child has their own temperament. Whereas some toddlers will have the occasional tantrum, others may have them regularly making it difficult for a parent to cope with them. However, they are a normal part of a child's development and happen for various reasons. It is thus imperative to tune in to your baby, stepping into the child's shoes to see why tantrums happen. Your child thinks he knows it all and does not need you. However, the realisation hits home that he is limited in knowledge and ability. He needs you to help him out but does not want to acknowledge it. He tries to do something, perhaps play with a toy that requires some problem solving. He can't solve it. The rational thing would be for him to ask for your help. But that would be admitting that he doesn't know everything. Plus, he wants an immediate solution. He decides to throw the toy on the floor in frustration and anger. The toy has the problem, not him. Sometimes, a toddler has a tantrum because he wants things done now. He wants your help with a task, but you ask him to wait. Then he explodes. He doesn't want to wait. Why should he? He is meant to be the centre of your life. And to him his problem is urgent, almost a matter of life and death. He demonstrates this urgency by a tantrum, which often gets a reaction from you.

A toddler may also have tantrums following the birth of a sibling. Prior to the birth of your baby, your toddler was the centre of attention. Now the new baby has come and stolen the show. He gets jealous and regresses to behaving like a baby to get attention. So if your newborn baby cries, your toddler feels the need to compete for your attention by crying louder and longer than your baby. If that doesn't work, he may resort to having a tantrum. Tantrums also happen when a child is tired, hungry or uncomfortable.

Another cause of tantrums is when you want your toddler to do something and he doesn't want to. You want your toddler to have his bath or change his nappy. He doesn't want to. According to him, he is his own master so why should he do what you want him to?

A further cause of tantrums is separation anxiety. Sometimes, parents go back to work when a child reaches toddlerhood, leaving the toddler feeling betrayed that you have 'abandoned' him. In anger, he throws a fit because he feels that you have left him with someone he doesn't love as much as you. Tantrums also happen as a result of a child's communication difficulties. A child may have difficulty expressing himself due to lack of language. He knows what he wants but can't express himself. As you try to guess, he loses patience with you and has a tantrum. From his own perspective, he is the centre of your life, so you should know what he wants at all times. He becomes frustrated and exhibits this in a tantrum. However, frustration is a part of a toddler's life as he learns about people, things and the way the world around him works, and that the world does not revolve around him. Thus, it is important for you to learn how to manage them.

> *'Tell me and I forget, teach me and I may remember, involve me and I learn.'*
>
> Benjamin Franklin, A founding father of the United States and polymath

How to Manage Tantrums

As always, I recommend tuning in to your baby. The management of a tantrum depends on your child's age, the cause of the behaviour and where the behaviour happens. The younger a child is, the less likelihood of rational thought being behind the behaviour. For example, a one-year-old child is less likely to think his actions through. He just acts. He wants something, wants it now, doesn't get it, tantrum! The way a parent manages the tantrum can however, determine how a child uses future tantrums. If a child gets the reaction he wants from the tantrum, it can be used as a weapon. The child says to himself, I got a reaction, I'll do that again! Thus, if not managed properly, as the child gets older he can use tantrums to his advantage, thinking them through and choosing the right moment such as a public place, or when you are in a rush to get the maximum effect.

I'm an avid believer of the prevention is better than cure approach. The best way to manage tantrums, knowing what causes them is to avoid them as much as possible. Ensure your child is getting enough attention from you to reduce the need for him to crave it and use his tantrums as a means of getting that attention. If you have just had a baby, it is important to spend time alone with your toddler to assure him that you still love him. Involve him in caring for his younger sibling so that he feels special. Send him on little errands, such as going to get his sibling's nappy and praise him when he successfully does so. Your child wants control of things, so try to give him some control over things by giving him some choices that you are happy to fulfil. As you get to know your child you will learn how to use choices. Some children are content with just two options, whereas other children need more. I soon realised as a parent that Joshua was not content with two options, the red socks or the blue socks. So sometimes I will give him five choices that I was happy with and this worked. When it came to changing his nappy, I had a changing unit where I would empty the pack of nappies. He loved choosing his own nappies even when the nappies all looked the same to me. When there were about three nappies left, I would have to open a new pack, because for Joshua, three nappies were not enough to choose from. I must stress that I am not suggesting that you need to bend over backwards to meet your child's needs for choice. I am just pointing out the need to work with your child. For me it was easier for me to have more nappies than to have a tantrum, especially if I was tired. As Joshua grew older, I made him understand that there will be times when there would be fewer options to choose from or only one choice. When they are older, this is easier to explain because they understand language and can express themselves.

As your child gets older, it is important to keep the home environment safe. Your child thinks that he knows everything as he has watched you doing things from the time he was born. As he grew, he wanted to copy what you did but was limited in ability. Now he is mobile, he can get to your things, for example the television or DVD player and he wants to copy what you do but has no understanding of risk. So you have to ensure he can explore safely. Keep off-limit things off limit! It will greatly reduce your need to say no, thus reducing the number of tantrums. It will also help prevent your child from having accidents. Of course, this is not always possible, especially outside your home.

Choose the times that you go out shopping or do other activities that can be tiresome for your toddler. If your child is tired or hungry it is not a good time to undertake these activities. When playing, understand your child's abilities. Offer age-appropriate toys to reduce the frustration your child may feel when playing with toys that overly challenge his ability. Imagine how it feels for him playing with his toy. When someone is trying to teach you a skill, you want them to make learning easy and enjoyable. You don't want them to start with the most difficult challenge. Do the same with your child, and he will enjoy learning and playing with you.

Communicate with your child. If your child wants to do something that you don't want him to do, explain the reasons why in a gentle, calm manner. Your toddler will not understand straight away, but over time he will learn that you mean what you say. Also, prepare your child for change. So if he is due to have a bath, give him a warning that his playtime will soon be over and he will be having a bath in five minutes. This gives your toddler the opportunity to wind down from one activity and prepare for the next.

Diversion is another useful technique. Your toddler has a short attention span, so use it! He wants something, but he can't have it. Find another thing that he likes or change his environment. He can't play with a particular object in the living room, so take him out to the garden or the park where he will find more interesting objects to play with.

Despite trying to prevent tantrums, there are times when your child will still have one. It is useful to remember that tantrums in themselves are not bad. A child needs to let off steam and express their emotions in a healthy way. It's the behaviours that accompany them such as biting, throwing his toys, and kicking, that you need to get rid of. Understand why tantrums happen but do not give in to them. If you show your child that you understand his feelings such as the frustration he is going through as he learns to express himself, it makes it easier to diffuse the tantrum. Your toddler needs to learn to manage his emotions and to express them in a healthy way.

But bad behaviours will not be rewarded. So be firm with telling your child that his inappropriate behaviour will not be tolerated. Your child needs to learn to handle difficult things, so stay with him. Doing so will reassure him that you are there for him but will also model for your child that you can handle the heat and not walk away at the first sign of trouble. If however, the tantrum worsens, and exhibits bad behaviour do not reward him with your attention. If you can look away and ignore him, do so and explain why you are doing so. If not, it may be time for time out. If your toddler wants your attention, he will have to behave well to get it. Giving your toddler time will allow him to cool down. Once he does, talk with him reaffirming that you love him but do not like his behaviour. Remember to label the act not the child. Tell him that he has done something naughty, not that he is a naughty child.

Parents dread tantrums especially in public places. But it is important for you not to let your toddler sense this. If he does, he may use it to his advantage. Try to prevent them by making sure your child is not tired or hungry. Toddlers like to help, so involve him as much as possible in the activity you are undertaking, for example if you are shopping. Each time he helps you, reward him with praise. If, despite all you do, he still has a tantrum, manage it the same way you would at home. If he persists, you may need to make a quick exit such as leaving the shop. He needs to learn he will not get attention, no matter how large the audience is.

If despite trying the above, you are still having problems with managing tantrums or your child's behaviour in general, do speak with your health visitor.

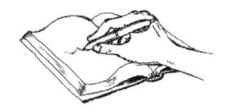

Please turn to the appendix and look for the heading *Planning for Tantrums.*

> *'Children are made readers on the laps of their parents.'*
> Emilie Buchwald, Author

Potty Training

Many parents often want to know when the best time to start potty training is. Every child is different and your child will only become potty trained when he is ready. Most children are physically and emotionally ready between two and two and a half years of age, with boys a bit later than girls. In the first 18 months, there is no proper bladder or bowel control. As such it is pointless starting this early. So wait at least until your child can walk or sit down and knows that he is wet or has a soiled nappy. There are also signs that your toddler may show you that he is ready to start toilet training. When he starts to imitate what you do in the toilet, such as pulling his pants down, wanting to sit on the toilet and wanting to flush the toilet for you, does not like the feeling of being wet or in a dirty nappy, can demonstrate that he wants to open his bowels, has words for urine and stools, has several dry nappies during the day, and shows a desire for independence.

Some parents also want to know whether they should potty train or toilet train. Although this is a matter of personal preference, there are advantages of using a potty over using the toilet. The potty is mobile and can be moved from room to room. If your toddler sees the potty, he is more likely to use it. It is also easier to use as some toddlers may have a fear of sitting on the toilet even if you get a toddler toilet seat. However, some toddlers prefer to sit on the toilet seat because that is what they see you doing. More important than the equipment used, is what you do and how you do it.

In order not to set your child up to fail, wait until your child is ready to be potty trained. Get a potty or a child toilet seat. If you want to use the toilet, you may want to get a child footstool so that your child can reach the toilet seat and steady their feet when they sit on the toilet seat. Get your child into the habit of sitting on the potty or toilet seat. Observe when your child usually opens his bowels and put him on the potty or toilet seat, fully clothed. If your child refuses to sit on the potty or toilet seat, do not force him. Just keep trying. If your child really doesn't want to sit on the potty or toilet, it may be a sign that he is not ready. So give him a break for about a month and try again. Keep trying until your child shows an interest. Once your child is interested, and you have got him into a routine of sitting on the toilet seat fully clothed, then your toddler is ready to try sitting on the toilet without a nappy. You may want to do this when you are using the toilet. Put the potty opposite you and as you pull your pants down, get your child to pull their nappy down too, and whilst you sit on the toilet, get him to sit on the potty. Again, if your child resists, do not force him. Let him just keep observing what you do. Eventually, he will copy what you do. Involve your child in the process and get him to see what you have done in the toilet and flush the toilet. Explain to him that his urine and stools will go in the potty or toilet and will have to be flushed away. Teach him to wash his hands after using the toilet. Encourage your toddler to use the potty or toilet as often as he needs to. If you can, allow him to walk around without a nappy so he can use the potty when he needs to. Whilst you can use pants, pull up and down training nappies will help you manage accidents that will inevitably happen. Most importantly, be consistent with what you do and persist at it. Reward your child with praise whenever he successfully uses the potty or toilet. You may also try using a reward or sticker chart. Remember that it's the little steps your toddler takes that add up to the journey! Accidents will happen so don't criticise your child for them. Just calmly clean the mess and encourage him to try to use the potty or toilet next time. Be patient and allow time for your child to learn. Eventually your child will be dry for most of the day and in due course at night too.

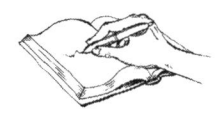

Please turn to the appendix and look for the heading *My Toddler Does Not Like the Potty.*

Communicate With Your Toddler

Communication is the lifeblood of any relationship. Thus, it is important that you communicate with your toddler. Your toddler is trying to make sense of the world around him but may have limited speech and expression. Therefore, it is important to continue to observe him. You can often tell what your toddler is trying to communicate by observing his body language. Babies and toddlers are very expressive and will use positive non-verbal language like smiles, laughs, cuddles and laughing to express their happiness with you and negative body language such as crying, grimacing, turning away, a tightened fist, or an upset look to express that they do not like an activity. Toddlers are quite impulsive and will often let you immediately know their feelings even if they don't have words to express clearly what they need. It is thus important that you do not only observe, but also respond as it is through exposure to speech and language that you toddler will learn to use language.

Promoting Speech

There are several things you can do to aid the development of your child's speech. Start by talking to him. If you have started talking and reading to your baby from pregnancy, it will now have become a habit and your toddler should be used to this. Continue to tell your toddler about everything you are doing, ensuring that you maintain good eye contact so that your child knows that he has your full attention. Observe his reaction to what you say, as this will determine your response. Continue to use every opportunity to teach your child how to speak. Bath time and when you are dressing your child are good times to teach your child about his body parts. Provide him the opportunity to repeat what you say and gently correct him when he does not get it right. When he does, praise him. When doing things for your toddler, offer him choices for him to learn language. So instead of just offering a cup, ask if he wants a red cup or a blue one, whilst pointing to each object. In that way, your child will not only learn the object is a cup, but will also get to learn colours. Whilst playing together, use verbal language. At this age, there is no need to use baby talk as your child needs to learn how to speak properly. What you teach your child is what he will learn. Playtime is a lovely opportunity to teach your child how to speak. So name his toys and describe them and get him to copy what you say. Whilst cooking, put him in a safe place next to you and tell him the names of the fruits, vegetables, and other foods you are cooking. Whilst eating, do the same. Whilst walking out and about, point out things of interest such as buses, cars, trains, stations, traffic lights, the red and green man, etc. Before long your toddler will develop and continue to grow his vocabulary. At about 8–12 months, your baby will start babbling and start to say words like dada or mama. It is important to note that a toddler understands more words than he can express. Therefore, at 18 months, your toddler understands about 50 words but may say about five; at 24 months, he will understand about 200–300 words, but may only say about 50; at three years he may know about 900 words but only use 300 frequently; and by four he will understand about 1,200 words but use 800 regularly. By two years of age, your toddler should be able to put two words together and will understand simple instructions. He'll also point to things he wants but can't express the word for. When he turns three, he'll be speaking in sentences and will use adjectives to describe things and can understand some prepositions, e.g. on, under, in, etc. If you are concerned about your child's speech or think your child has a speech delay please contact your health visitor.

It is also important to talk to your toddler and listen to his feelings. Let your child express his feelings of joy, sadness, anger, frustration, fear and respond to them. Try and feel how your child feels and let him know that it is all right to feel these feelings and that you sometimes feel that way too. Whilst doing this, it is important to use language that your toddler understands and gestures may help you to communicate this to your child. It may also help if you repeat the words that your child has used and employ good eye contact to show that you are listening and check that you understand what your child said. Encourage your child to say more by not interrupting him. Reassure him that you're listening by using expressions such as 'yeah . . .', 'ok. . .', 'really. . .', 'tell me more. . .' And if he has done wrong, do not blame him, but explain to him the reason why what he has done was not right and why you don't want him to repeat this. Remember that your toddler may not understand everything that you say. It is a gradual and continuous process for your child to learn, and you as a parent will require a lot of patience. But the rewards are great, especially when you observe your toddler telling others not to do something that he once used to do and explains the reason why.

Speak with your child about things that matter to you such as your culture, your faith and similar important things as he will grow up with these. I remember having to call my dad, granddad; and my mum, grandma; as Joshua just repeated what I called them and was calling my dad, dad; and my mum, mum. Over time, Joshua eventually learned to call them granddad and grandma, because that was what I called them. Being an African, respect is important and as such a young child can't refer to an older person by their first name. Thus, I had to call my brothers Uncle Nick, and Uncle Michael and put aunty and uncle titles before all my friends' names. I did not want Joshua to refer to them by their first names, as it is often seen as rude in my culture. I also taught him to say a proper greeting such as good morning, afternoon or evening, rather than *hi* or *hello*, as casual greetings from a young child to an older person is also deemed rude in my culture.

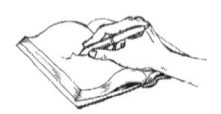

Please turn to the appendix and look for the heading *Teaching My Toddler.*

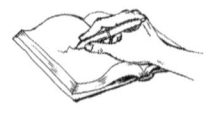

Please turn to the appendix and look for the heading *Playing with My Toddler.*

TUNE IN TO YOUR BABY

> *'What it's like to be a parent: it's one of the hardest things you'll ever do but in exchange it teaches you the meaning of unconditional love.'*
>
> Nicholas Sparks, Novelist and screenwriter

There's No Point Saying 'No!'

As a parent you may get frustrated when you say no to your toddler because your toddler just ignores you and goes ahead and does what you didn't want them to anyway. Although some babies may understand what no means at about six months, most babies will go ahead and ignore it until they are about 12–18 months. The more you say it, the more it will be ignored as your baby may not understand what you mean and just repeat it and smile, thinking it is a game. Therefore it is better to use words that make clear the reason why you want your toddler to stop or avoid what it is you they want to do. For example, rather than say no when a toddler is about to touch something hot, say 'hot' or 'hurt you'. The tone of voice that you use will also send an alarm to your child not to do it. Before I realised this, despite baby-proofing the house and ensuring it was safe enough to explore his surroundings, Joshua was sometimes interested in getting to things that were more attractive than his toys. He preferred the television and would stand just in front of it and try to press the buttons. When I would tell him no, he would repeat it and even repeat my gestures, pointing his little finger at me. He almost appeared to do so simultaneously as I did. He knew what to expect and anticipated it. It was as if he was thinking, I want to do what mummy does, and she is going to say no. I know this and I will just copy her. And he would laugh as he did this, thinking it was a game. Eventually, I realised that saying no all the time was not working and had to change tactic.

While your conscious brain can understand negatives, there is some evidence that the subconscious mind does not understand negatives and as such ignores them. This is why toddlers often do the opposite of what they are told to do. So when you tell your toddler not to do something, they delete the word *not* and then do it, because that is what they've heard you say. For example, you tell your toddler not to touch something and then he touches it. You think he is defiant, but he actually doesn't understand what you said. He gets told off by you leaving him confused. He thinks he has done what you asked and so cannot understand why you are cross. It can be difficult turning negative statements into positive ones, but with practise it can be done and it will enable your toddler to understand what you mean.

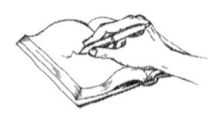

Please turn to the appendix and look for the heading *Positive Talk*.

> 'Your kids require you most of all to love them for who they are, not to spend your whole time trying to correct them.'
>
> Bill Ayer, American elementary education theorist

What Kind of Parent Are You?

Whilst managing toddler behaviour can be challenging, your parenting style can influence how your toddler behaves and can make it easier or more difficult to manage his behaviour. Research done in the early 1960s by psychologist Diana Baumrind and further developed in the 1980s by Maccoby and Martin identified four main parenting styles.

Authoritarian Parent – high control, low acceptance and nurture

This type of parent likes to control their toddler and is less accepting of his behaviour. Such a parent adopts a very strict 'do as I say' approach without allowing the toddler a voice. Authoritarian parents also set many rules and monitor their children ensuring their children abide by them whilst offering little or no emotional support. The toddler may initially resist his parent's approach, but the parent asserts more force and power, until the child learns submission and not to question things. As a result he may become passive and anxious when the parent is around. Whilst this may work for a period of time, eventually the child would gain freedom and is more likely to rebel against a lot of what he has been taught as he was never given an opportunity to exercise choice.

Permissive Parent – low control, high acceptance and nurture

The permissive parent is the opposite of the authoritarian parent. Such a parent does not control their toddler, is highly supportive and sets few rules and does not monitor if rules are followed. Instead permissive parents trust their children. They are very indulgent, can't say no and stick to it, are anxious to please their children and are easily manipulated. It is almost as if the parent and child roles are reversed. As a result the toddler tends to have high expectations of the parent and become very demanding of them. They are also easily frustrated as they become impatient with what appears to be their parents 'slow' response to their needs. This parenting style can create problems for toddlers as they have little understanding of the world around them. Such a child will grow up to be self-centred, spoilt, and expect that everything happens the way that they want.

Passive Parent – low control, low acceptance and nurture

The passive parent is neglectful. Passive parents adopt a 'learn from your mistakes' approach, offering no guidance for their toddlers. They set no rules and just expect the child to get on with it. They prioritise their needs over the child's needs and give very little attention to their children. They will focus mainly on the child's physical needs and pay no attention to their child's emotional needs. They don't demand anything from their toddler, neither do they regulate him. They do not show they love their children, neither do they discipline them. A toddler of a neglectful parent is likely to grow up detached, or insecurely attached and may have difficulty forming relationships as they have not learned to trust their main care provider from an early age. He tends to have little self-control and poor social skills.

Authoritative Parent – high control, high acceptance and nurture

The authoritative parent balances control with acceptance and nurture. Such a parent balances love and discipline, and regards their child as unique They set boundaries for him. They respect their children and will reward them with privileges when earned. They are firm, will use reasoning, and encourage independence. Authoritative parents will allow their children to question them and provide guidance and support. Even when they use discipline, it is supportive rather than punitive. Children of authoritative parents are happy, well regulated, self-motivated, cooperative, and confident.

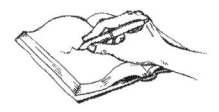

> Please turn to the appendix and look for the heading *What is My Choice of Parenting Style?*

Managing Toddler Behaviour

In view of the above, the authoritative approach seems to be the best parenting style for raising children, especially toddlers. You can become such a parent if you tune in to your baby's needs. The toddler years can be a frustrating time for your child. Therefore, work with your child to understand his frustration. Contain his emotions whilst he learns to manage them. Set very clear boundaries with your toddler, so he knows what you expect of him. The key to managing toddler behaviour is consistency and persistence. It may take a while for your child to understand what you say, but be consistent and persistent. Repetition will help embed the learning. As your toddler grows, give him some more independence. Offer your child options to give them some control. Reward his good behaviour with treats and privileges such as star charts. When he does not behave well, take these away. Over time, you toddler will come to understand he is responsible for his actions and can control them.

Apart from your parenting style, I must also stress that you and your partner are consistent in parenting your toddler. If your toddler senses that you are not in unison, he may use it to his advantage and try to manipulate either of you to his advantage. Thus, it is imperative that you raise and discipline your toddler together. Even though Joshua's dad and I don't live together, we regularly discussed Joshua's needs and worked together to manage the toddler years. Even though Joshua spent some weekends at his dad's house, his routine was maintained making it easier to keep his home routine. Despite this Joshua still tried to play us against each other. He would sometimes tell his dad that he was allowed to do some things such as sleep later, consume fizzy drinks, etc. But his dad would make a telephone call to me to confirm if this was true. Once Joshua realised that he could not play us against each other, this behaviour stopped.

Love and Manage Yourself

Sometimes, it is not the toddler's behaviour that is not right, but our tolerance of his behaviour. Some toddler behaviour is normal but as parents, we are occasionally tired and can't handle it. As such it is important to look after and manage yourself. When your toddler behaves in an inappropriate manner the initial reaction may be to snap at him showing him how angry you are with his behaviour. If you are stressed, he may use this to his advantage and push your buttons even more. It is important to respond and not just react. Choose the response that is most likely to create the outcome you want. Remain calm but firm. In that way, you will be modelling how you want your child to act when he is angry. Once your child has calmed down, discuss the reason for his behaviour and administer discipline.

The human brain is a negative feedback loop system. As such, rather than noticing what is right, your brain focuses on what is wrong: a mismatch, with a view to adjusting it. For example, when you are hungry, there is a mismatch and your brain sends signals for you to correct hunger. You then feel the need to eat in order to correct the hunger. You eat and are satisfied and feel happy and return to normal. When everything is all right in the body, there is no mismatch and no feedback is given. The same can happen with our interactions with our toddlers. Rather than noticing the good they do, we can pick up on the negative that they do. Most of the time (about 80 per cent), your child behaves well and it is only about 20 per cent of the time that he misbehaves. It is very easy to forget all the good times the child behaves and remember the occasions that he behaves inappropriately. It is thus crucial to focus on the very many times that your toddler behaves, showering him with praise for his conduct. It may encourage him to keep his good behaviour up.

Learn to love yourself and accept who you are. Wake up each morning, look in the mirror and tell yourself the reasons why you love yourself. Be kind to yourself and do not become over critical of what you do. Celebrate yourself and your achievements. Count your blessings. Instead of looking at the half empty glass, focus on the half full glass. When you stagnate, it can get you down. Therefore, set goals and commit to action as it will boost your confidence. Endeavour to plan every day that you live, and celebrate and fix it at the end. When you love yourself, it is easier for your child and others around you to love you. Your child will come to know what love is and be more likely to reciprocate it.

Love Your Toddler

Let your toddler know how much you love him. This is important especially when you discipline him. Although discipline may not feel like it, it is an act of love. It is often said that love is not love until it is expressed. So show your toddler how much you love him through displays of affection. Reaffirm it with words. Make time for him so that he does not have to resort to negative behaviour to earn your attention. Reward him with praise and compliments. Love and manage yourself so that you can tune in to your baby's needs.

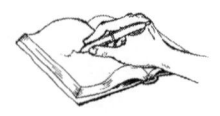

Please turn to the appendix and look for the heading *My Special Toddler.*

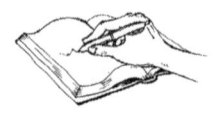

Please turn to the appendix and look for the heading *Love for Yourself, Toddler and Others.*

Sharing My Learning

- Although managing the toddler years can be challenging, you can handle them.
- Tune in to your toddler to try to understand why he behaves the way he does.
- Your toddler wants to be independent, so offer him options to give him some control.
- Communicate with your toddler regularly using positive statements, as your toddler's brain cannot process negative statements.
- Work with your toddler to manage the challenges he may face.
- Be patient, consistent and persistent.
- Your parenting style can affect your toddler's behaviour. Endeavour to adopt an authoritative approach.
- An authoritative approach is where control is balanced with acceptance and nurture.
- Work with your partner to establish clear boundaries for your toddler. Jointly agree how you will discipline your toddler and enforce it.
- Love and manage yourself in order to be able to love and manage your toddler.

> *'Children have never been very good at listening to their elders, but they have never failed to imitate them.'*
>
> James Baldwin, American novelist, essayist, playwright, poet, and social critic

Chapter 6

Putting It All Into Practice

Looking back I can't believe how much I have grown. I have learned a lot from my experiences of pregnancy, childbirth and parenting. I can honestly say that Joshua is the best thing that has happened to me. He has taught me so much about myself and parenting. My parenting journey has not been easy but the rewards have been immense. I have learned first *how not to* parent Joshua before learning *how to* parent him. I have learned to tune in to him to discern his needs. Now it's much easier as he can use language to express his needs.

It is often said that knowledge brings with it power. I would state that this is not always true. We as adults know so many things. However, we don't always act on that knowledge. What I have found empowers you is **action**, i.e. acting on the knowledge you have. I would like to share an equation that I've found very useful and that has enabled my growth. It is:

BE	+	DO	=	HAVE
Who you are BEING	+	**What you are DOING**	=	**What you HAVE**

Put simply, who you choose to be as a parent empowers you to do things that will lead you to having the results you get.

So if you want to have a happy child, you have to *choose* to be happy as a parent, and do the things that will enable you to have a happy child. Note, that I use the word *choose*. We sometimes may not realise that we have chosen the things we have. Pause for a second and think: why is it that two different individuals can experience exactly the same thing under the same circumstances and have different results? It's all down to who they choose to be and what they do. I recognised this in pregnancy when things were not going my way. It was very easy to blame anyone but myself for how things were unfolding, especially as I experienced setback after setback. As soon as I decided to take responsibility and used my ability to choose my response – managed my thoughts, feelings and actions, I was able to tune in to my baby in order find out his needs, and meet them. So can you!

In pregnancy, childbirth and parenting there are so many things out of our control. However, there are also many things that are within our control. You have total control of your mind, who you choose to be, and what you choose to do. Your choices will determine your results – what you will have.

Included throughout this book are useful tips that you can try that will help you tune in to your baby, find out what his needs are and successfully meet them. However, knowing is not enough. Action is required. Make it your responsibility to tune in to your baby and enjoy parenting from the time your baby is conceived until your baby has the ability to use language to express his needs. Be committed to looking after you, your baby and those that matter to you. Be consistent with whatever you do and be persistent, as it will eventually pay off. Every day will be a learning experience, but you will grow as you learn and be ready for the next chapter as a parent.

Whilst this book is packed with lots of information about how to tune in to your baby, it has its limitations like any other book. It is not comprehensive and has not covered all aspects of parenting. That is why I urge you to attend one my workshops and/or live webinars where you will be able to connect with other parents and go into greater depth than the book is able to and explore the parenting issues that are pertinent to you. At these workshops and webinars, we will be able to use interactive exercises and shared expertise to enable you to learn to parent your baby successfully. I am looking forward to connecting with you soon.

More information is available at *www.tuneintoyourbaby.com*

> *'Mother is a verb. It's something you do.*
> *Not just who you are.'*
>
> Cheryl Lacey Donovan, Author and evangelist

Important Notice

Seeking professional support to help you manage stress and emotions is a good idea. Sometimes, all it takes is the helping hand of a knowledgeable, caring professional to help motivate or support you, so you can start coping again. Sadly, some people do not find it easy to seek help. But just as our bodies need to get help from the doctor when we feel unwell, sometimes our mind deserves help too.

Please seek immediate help if you are experiencing any of the following:

- Thoughts of death or suicide.
- Negative, or self-destructive, thoughts you cannot control.
- Using alcohol, food, or drugs, to help control difficult emotions.
- Feeling helpless, despair, and hopeless, most of the time.
- Chronic difficulty sleeping.
- Lack of ability to concentrate, to the point where it is affecting your work or home life.

The Samaritans:

www.samaritans.org

| UK | 08457 909090 |
| ROI | 1850 609090 |

Mind - The leading mental health charity for England & Wales
www.mind.org.uk
0300 1233393

NHS Direct - Offers health advice and reassurance 24hours a day, 365 days a year.
England and Wales: 0845 4647
Scotland: 08454 242424

Bibliography and References

Bradford, M. (2009) *Transcending The Victim-Rescuer-Persecutor Triangle*. Available at: http://www.holisticworld.co.uk/your_say.php?article_id=77

Bowlby, J. (1988) *A Secure Base.* Routledge, London.

Byrd, A. (1988) *The Power of Touch*. Available at: http://www.goodhousekeeping.com/health/wellness/health-benefits-of-touch

Chapman, A. (2006) *Elisabeth Kübler-Ross – Five Stages of Grief*. Available at: www.businessballs.com/elisabeth_kubler_ross_five_stages_of_grief.htm

Childbirth Graphics (2003) Growing a Baby. Available at: www.childbirthgraphics.com

Chitty, A., Mischenko, J., Johnson, J., Ranger, S. (2007) *Understanding Your Baby*, Leeds Primary Care Trust.

Collins English Dictionary (2009) Complete & Unabridged 10th Edition. William Collins Sons & Co. Ltd.

Council of Europe (2002). *Recommendation of the Committee of Ministers to member States on the protection of women against violence.* Adopted on 30 April 2002 ; and *Explanatory Memorandum*. (Strasbourg, France Council of Europe).

Covey, S. R. (2004) *The Seven Habits of Highly Effective People. Powerful Lessons in Personal Change.* 15th edition. Simon and Schuster, London:

Department of Health (2009a) *The Pregnancy Book.* Available at: www.dh.gov.uk/prod_consum_dh/ groups/dh_digitalassets/@dh/@en/@ps/@sta/@perf/ documents/digitalasset/dh_117166.pdf

Department of Health (2009b) *Birth to Five.* Available at: www.dh.gov.uk/en/Publicationsandstatistics/ Publications/PublicationsPolicyAndGuidance/ DH_107303

Dispenza, J. (2007) *Evolve Your Brain.* Health Communications Inc., Florida

Ellison, K. (2005) *The Mommy Brain: How Motherhood Makes Us Smarter.* Basics Books, NY

Gerhardt, S. (2004) *Why Love Matters: How affection shapes a babies brain.* Routledge, Hove.

Green, C. (2003) *Toddler Taming Tips: A Parent's Guide to the First Four Years.* Vermilion, London.

Green, C. (2006) *New Toddler Taming: A Parent's Guide to the First Four Years.* Vermilion, London.

Jeffers, S. (1991) *Feel the Fear and Do It Anyway.* Arrow, London.

Kübler-Ross, E. (1969) *On Death and Dying,* Macmillan, New York.

Lim, O. (2005) *Prenatal Stimulation For A Smart Baby.* Available at: www.ezinearticles.com/?Prenatal-Stimulation-For-A-Smart-Baby&id=76513

Mayne, B. *Goal Mapping: The Practical Workbook. How to Turn Your Dreams into Realities.* Watkins Publishing, London.

Mayo Clinic *Pregnancy week by week Fetal development: The second trimester* Available at: www.mayoclinic.com/health/fetal-development/PR00113

Melton, K. (2010) *Trauma Caused By 'Emergency' & 'Failure to Progress' C-Sections to Mom & Baby. In Prevention of Healing and Womb, Birth and Bonding Trauma.* Accessed at: www.healyourearlyimprints.com/blog on 12th May 2012.

Mohrbacher, N., Stock, J., (2003) *La Leche League International. The Breast-feeding Answer Book.* La Leche League International, Illinois.

Murray L., and Andrews L. (2005) *The Social Baby: Understanding Babies' Communication from Birth.* Richmond: CP Publishing.

Newman, J. (2009) *The Importance of Skin to Skin Contact* Accessed at: www.nbci.ca/index.php?option=com_content&view=article&id=82:the-importance-of-skin-to-skin-contact-&catid=5:information&Itemid=17

The Nemours Foundation (2012) *Bonding with Your Baby.* Accessed at www.kidshealth.org/parent/pregnancy_newborn/communicating/bonding.html#

NSPCC/Children's Project (2004) *The Social Baby: Understanding Babies' Communication from Birth (DVD)*. Available at: www.nspcc.org.uk

Oshikanlu, R. (2012) *My Baby Manual: Because Babies Don't Come with An Instruction Manual*. 90 Day Books, England

Peterson, G. (1999) *What is 'good enough' parenting?* Available at: www.ivillage.com

Rankin, C. *The motherhood blues* Available at: www.yourparenting.co.za/family/my-time/being-a-mom/the-motherhood-blues

Robinson, M. (2010) *Infant Mental Health: Effective prevention and early intervention*. Unite/CPHVA

Robinson, L., Saisan, L., Smith, M., Segal, J. (2012) *Building a Secure Attachment Bond With Your Baby: Parenting Tips for creating a strong attachment relationship*. Available at: www.helpguide.org/mental/parenting_attachment.htm

Ronberg, G. (2010) *Baby Brain Development in the Womb* Available at: www.livestrong.com/article/207982-baby-brain-development-in-the-womb

Serendip (2008) *The Effects of Sleep Deprivation on Brain and Behavior*. Available at: www.serendip.brynmawr.edu

Snelson, J. C. (2006) *Pre-Birth Communication and Bonding*. Available at: www.unhinderedliving.com/prebirthbonding.html

Solomon, C. (2003) *Transactional Analysis Theory: the Basics. Transactional Analysis Journal 33 (1): 15 - 22*

Staff, T. (2012) *The Value of Playing With Your Child.* Available at: www.thecutekid.com/parenting/parents-playing-children.php

Sunderland, M. (2007) *What Every Parent Needs to Know: The incredible effects of love, nurture and play on your child's development.* Dorling Kindersley, London.

The Baby Friendly Initiative (2011) *Breast-feeding.* Available at: www.unicef.org.uk

Tommys; *Premature Birth Statistics.* Available at: www.tommys.org/page.aspx?pid=387

Unite/CPHVA (2012) *Managing Colic. Community Practitioner Educational Supplement.* Vol. 15.

UI Maternity Centre (2004) *Understanding Your Baby's Signals.* Available at: www.uihealthcare.com

Online References and Useful Websites

Expert advice on feeding toddlers.
www.infantandtoddlerforum.org

The UK's biggest parenting website with unique local information.
www.netmums.com

Current medical information and news on health topics provided by Clinical experts.
www.mayoclinic.com

UK based discussion forum offering support and companionship for pregnancy and early years of parenting.
www.babyworld.co.uk/

Online resource for new and expectant parents.
www.babycentre.co.uk

For information about holistic approach to birth preparation.
www.birthingfromwithin.com

For information about attachment and bonding.
www.helpguide.org/mental/parenting_attachment.htm

For information about the grief cycle.
www.changingminds.org/disciplines/change_management/kubler_ross/kubler_ross.htm

www.businessballs.com/elisabeth_kubler_ross_five_stages_of_grief.htm

For more information about naming traditions in Africa.
www.mercatornet.com/articles/view/names_and_the_value_of_a_human_person

For more information about how habits are formed.
www.truehealthandhealing.org/how-habits-are-formed-in-the-nervous-system.html

For more information about nesting.
www.parentingweekly.com/pregnancy/pregnancy-symptoms/nesting-instinct.htm

Online resource for children's health and development.
www.kidshealth.org/parent/growth/senses/sensenewborn.html#

Online resource that provides useful sleep advice for children's health and development.
www.baby-sleep-advice.com/why-is-sleep-important.html#ixzz1uktZYln1

For more information on sleep and sleep cycles.
www.helpguide.org/life/sleeping.htm

For more information about domestic abuse and support for women and children that have experienced domestic violence.
www.womensaid.org.uk/domestic-violence-articles.asp?section=0001001002200410001&itemid=1272

For information about dealing with loneliness in motherhood.
www.askamum.co.uk/Mum/Search-Results/Relationships/Loneliness-in-motherhood-/

Transcript of Steve Jobs commencement speech for Stanford University.

www.blinksoflife.tumblr.com/post/779983497/steve-jobs-commencement-speech-for-stanford

The Drama Triangle.
www.mental-health-today.com/articles/drama.htm

Managing Parental Guilt.
www.life.familyeducation.com/parenting/self-image/45339.html#ixzz1vTQ9QuZ0

For more information about managing excessively crying babies.
www.cry-sis.org.uk

For more information about calming a crying baby.
www.problemshared.info

For more information about breastfeeding support.
www.breastfeedingnetwork.org.uk

About The Author

Ruth Oshikanlu has a professional background that spans 20 years working in different clinical and community settings as a nurse, midwife and health visitor. She previously worked on the Family Nurse Partnership – a nurse-led intensive home visiting programme commissioned by the Department of Health as part of the social exclusion plan to improve the life chances of pregnant teenagers and their babies. She supported vulnerable, hard to reach families, building therapeutic relationships and addressing complex family issues. Ruth utilised a strengths-based, solution-focused approach to enable clients and their families to improve their health and wellbeing, promote behaviour change, develop self-efficacy and reduce health inequalities. She is a single parent and is passionate about parenting. Her special interests include breast-feeding, infant mental health, and delivering parenting programmes.

Ruth is also a professional life coach and Goal Mapping Practitioner and has a passion for enabling others to achieve their full potential. She recognises the vast potential of human capability and understands what restrains this and how to unleash it. She has worked with several clients assisting them in identifying strengths and areas for improvement in a positive way, helping them to set clear and compelling goals, and empowering them to create innovative solutions. She is known for her warmth, humour and energy as well as her passion for creating a climate in which to maximise learning.

Appendix – My Baby Manual

This appendix is a toolkit to help you create your own baby manual. It is also available as an A4-sized companion book: *My Baby Manual: Because Babies Don't Come with An Instruction Manual* (Oshikanlu, 2012).

My Baby's Name

Contents

Finding Out That You Are Expecting a Baby A-1
How Do I Feel About Being Pregnant? A-4
Calculating Baby's Due Date A-5
My Baby's First Picture A-5
Tune In To My Growth Inside Your Womb A-6
    First Three Months (Weeks 1 – 13) A-6
    Second Three Months (Weeks 14 – 27) A-7
    Last Three Months (Weeks 28 – 40) A-8
My Baby's Picture – At 20 weeks A-9
Naming My Baby A-10
Baby and Me Time A-12
Planning My Baby's Birth A-14
How Do I Feel About Becoming a Mum? A-16
Prepare To Enjoy Motherhood A-17
My Day Now! A-18
My Day After Baby's Here! A-19
Feel Your Baby's Journey in to the World A-20
Mimic the Womb, Outside the Womb A-22
Your Baby's Cues A-22
Your Baby's States A-23
Contain Your Baby's Emotions A-23
Breast-feeding Your Baby - How is it going? A-26
Love for You, Baby and Others A-28
Playing With Your Baby A-30
How Do I Feel About Being A Mum? A-31
How Does It Feel To Be a Mum? A-32
Celebrate Motherhood! A-34
Where Are You in The Learning Circle? A-36
Making Adult Decisions A-38
    Choice of Feeding A-38
    Choice of Childcare A-39
My Special Baby: A-40
Could It Be Colic? A-41

Teaching My Baby	A-44
Find Your 20 Per Cent	A-46
My Daily Planner	A-49
Managing My Feelings	A-70
Breaking My Thinking Pattern	A-72
I'm Going Back to Work – Plan For Success!	A-74
Why the Guilt?	A-76
Home and Work Swap	A-78
More Loving, Playing and Learning	A-79
How Much Sleep Does My Toddler Get?	A-81
My Toddler's Food Diary	A-82
Planning for Tantrums	A-83
My Toddler Does Not Like the Potty	A-85
Teaching My Toddler	A-86
Playing With My Toddler	A-88
Positive Talk	A-89
What is My Choice of Parenting Style?	A-91
My Special Toddler	A-92
Love For Yourself, Toddler and Others	A-93

TUNE IN TO YOUR BABY: APPENDIX

Finding Out That You Are Expecting a Baby

Pregnancy, labour, and childbirth are all unpredictable events in life. Even when we plan for them, we do not have total control over the events that happen. We do however; have total control over our reaction to all the unpredictable events that happen at these times. It works like this:

Unpredictable Event	plus your	**Reaction**	creates the	**Outcome**
(E)		**(R)**		**(O)**

Our reaction to whatever events we experience in pregnancy, childbirth, labour can affect the outcome we get. So in order to influence the outcome, to get what we want, we need to react in a particular way. We do have control over thoughts, feelings and actions. Further, the way we think, affects the way we feel and thus our actions. For example, if we want to act in a positive way, we would need to think in a positive way, which will enable us to feel positive and thus act positively!

This manual should help you to process your thoughts and feelings, which may enable you to choose your actions more appropriately. It can empower you to tune in to your baby so you can determine what his/her needs may be. As you go through, be determined to enjoy creating your Baby Manual, tuning in to your baby's needs and parenting your baby.

When a woman finds out that she is pregnant, one of the things she does is share the news. The way that you feel about being pregnant affects you and your baby. The way others react to the news affects the way you feel and thus the way you feel about your baby. It is important to be nurtured at this time if you are to nurture your baby. Here are a few questions that can help you process your feelings about being pregnant. Answering them can also help you in developing your support networks.

What was your first thought when you found out that you were pregnant?

....

....

....

How did you feel?

....

....

....

....

What did you do?

....
....
....
....
....

Whom did you first tell?

....
....
....

What was their reaction?

....
....
....

How did it make you feel?

....
....
....

What are you going to do to ensure that you enjoy the rest of your pregnancy?

....
....
....
....
....

TUNE IN TO YOUR BABY: APPENDIX

....
....
....
....
....

Who is going to support your pregnancy and in what way?

....
....
....
....
....
....
....
....
....

Remember that you can also get professional support. So speak with your doctor or midwife.

How Do I Feel About Being Pregnant? – Pregnancy Gains and Losses

Pregnancy Gains: Things that I love about being pregnant

....
....
....
....
....
....
....
....
....
....

Pregnancy Losses: Things that I have lost because I am pregnant

....
....
....
....
....
....
....
....
....
....
....

TUNE IN TO YOUR BABY: APPENDIX

Calculating Baby's Due Date

Finding out when baby is due can help you plan for pregnancy and childbirth. You can calculate this before you see a midwife as follows:

- Write the first day of your last menstrual period (LMP): ....
- Then add one year to that date: ....
- Take away three months: ....
- Add seven days: ....

Baby's estimated date of delivery is:..

Remember this is only an estimate. Your due date will be confirmed or corrected at the dating scan. Also, normal pregnancy is between 37-42 weeks. Therefore, your baby may be born before or after your due date.

My Baby's First Picture

Paste a copy of your baby's dating scan picture here

RUTH OSHIKANLU

Tune In To My Growth Inside Your Womb

I am your baby. Below is the timeline of how I will grow in your womb. I want you to tune in to what is happening to me in your womb. There are two columns below. The first column is blank. Put a tick in each box at the beginning of each week of your pregnancy. It gives you and me a feeling of progression. The second column has an unborn baby in a heart. This represents me in your womb floating in abundant love. I want you to close your eyes and imagine how I am growing inside of you and what parts of me are developing.

Put a tick inside each baby at the end of each week of pregnancy if you have been able to tune in to me growing inside of you. This may be hard at first, but should become a habit over time. Enjoy following my growth and development inside your womb.

First Three Months (Weeks 1 – 13)

Gestation In weeks	✓	What is Happening to Me Inside Your womb	✓
Week 1	☐	First day of last menstrual period (LMP)	🤍
Week 2	☐	Ovulation and conception	🤍
Week 3	☐	Implantation	🤍
Week 4	☐	Missed period – often when most women discover that they may be pregnant	🤍
Week 5	☐	My central nervous system is forming	🤍
Week 6	☐	My brain, arms, legs and major organs are forming	🤍
Week 7	☐	My eyes are forming and muscles developing	🤍
Week 8	☐	My face is developing, ear structure and bones forming	🤍
Week 9	☐	My tooth buds are formed, I start to move but you can't feel me just yet	🤍
Week 10	☐	My lungs are developing and my heart is functioning at a basic level	🤍

TUNE IN TO YOUR BABY: APPENDIX

Week	11	☐	My head is about half of my total body length
Week	12	☐	My neck, mouth and nose are developing, my toes and fingers are formed
Week	13	☐	The placenta that nourishes me is completely formed

Second Three Months (Weeks 14 – 27)

Gestation In weeks		✓	What is Happening to Me Inside Your womb	✓
Week	14	☐	My genitals are developing	
Week	15	☐	I may suck my thumb	
Week	16	☐	Lanugo (fine, downy hair) is forming on my skin, which serves as insulation for me as I do not have fat layers. My body is growing quickly	
Week	17	☐	My fingernails and toenails are growing	
Week	18	☐	My heartbeat can be easily heard with a foetal heart monitor. If I'm a girl, my ovaries are developing	
Week	19	☐	You should start feeling me moving, stretching and kicking	
Week	20	☐	My scalp hair is growing	
Week	21	☐	My skin is very thin with little or no fat layers underneath	
Week	22	☐	My eyebrows and eyelashes are developing	
Week	23	☐	My head is about a third of my total body length. My fingerprints and toe prints are developing and my body is covered in lanugo (fine, downy hair) to keep me warm and vernix (a waxy coating that helps protect me from the amniotic fluid, moisturise my skin and prevent me from getting infections)	
Week	24	☐	I am gaining weight rapidly	
Week	25	☐	If I am born now, I may be able to survive with specialist help	

Week	26	☐	My lungs are developing but are still immature	
Week	27	☐	My eyebrows and eyelashes are fully developed	

Last Three Months (Weeks 28 – 40)

Gestation In weeks		✓	What is Happening to Me Inside Your womb	✓
Week	28	☐	My brain tissue is increasing	
Week	29	☐	My eyes are able to open, close and blink. My fat layers are developing	
Week	30	☐	I am practising breathing	
Week	31	☐	I should settle into the head-down position between now and my birth	
Week	32	☐	My organs continue to mature	
Week	33	☐	My lungs are nearing maturity	
Week	34	☐	Most of my body systems are well developed	
Week	35	☐	I can respond to familiar voices	
Week	36	☐	My kidneys are mature	
Week	37	☐	I have a firm grasp reflex	
Week	38	☐	My head is about a quarter of my total body length. My growth rate is slowing down	
Week	39	☐	My bones are fully formed and my lungs are mature. The lanugo and vernix on my body is disappearing. I may settle into a quiet period.	
Week	40	☐	I am now full term, i.e. 9 months, 40 weeks, or 280 days old. If I am not born yet, then expect me anytime now. I am ready to see your face!	

Adapted from Growing a Baby (Childbirth Graphics, 2003)

TUNE IN TO YOUR BABY: APPENDIX

My Baby's Picture – At 20 weeks

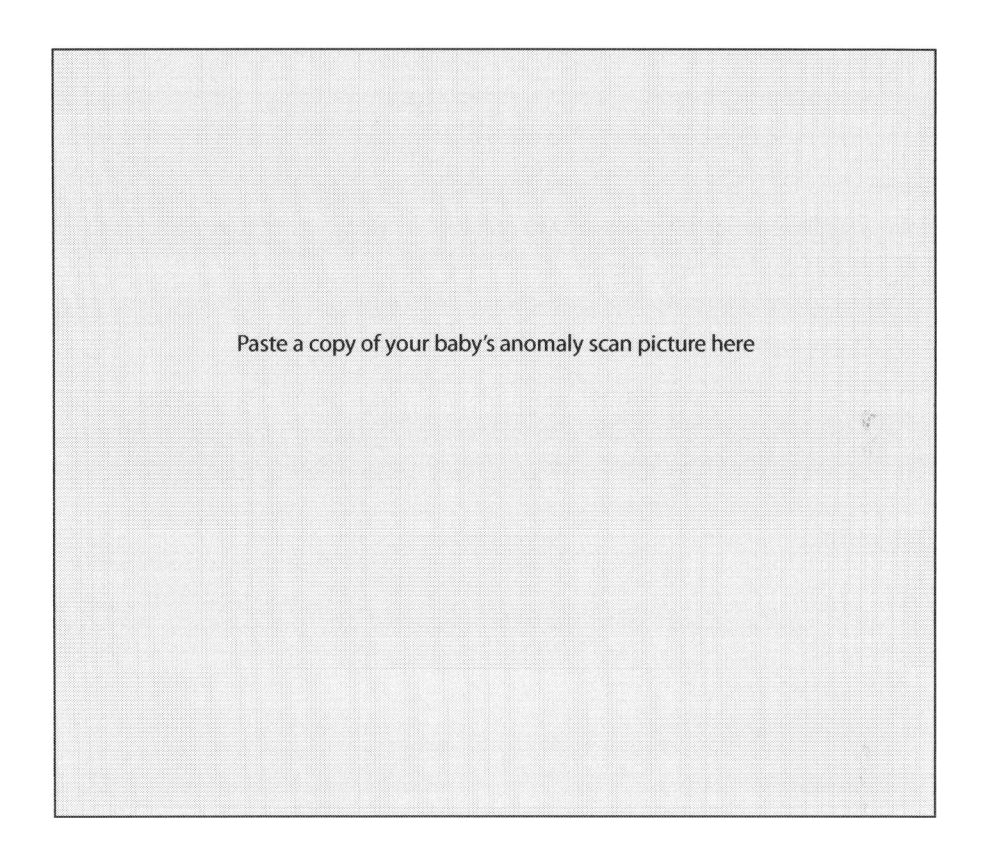

Paste a copy of your baby's anomaly scan picture here

RUTH OSHIKANLU

Naming My Baby

If my baby is a boy, what name(s) will I give him? Why?

Name .... Why?..

....

....

Name .... Why?..

....

....

Name .... Why?..

....

....

Name .... Why?..

....

....

Name .... Why?..

....

....

Name .... Why?..

....

....

....

TUNE IN TO YOUR BABY: APPENDIX

If my baby is a girl, what name(s) will I give her? Why?

Name .... Why?..
....
....

Name .... Why?..
....
....

Name .... Why?..
....
....

Name .... Why?..
....
....

Name .... Why?..
....
....

Name .... Why?..
....
....
....

Baby and Me Time

When do you sit and spend time with your Baby?
....

How long does it last?
....
....

What do you do?
....
....
....
....
....
....

How does baby respond?
....
....
....
....

What does s/he like?
....
....
....

TUNE IN TO YOUR BABY: APPENDIX

What does s/he dislike?

....
....
....
....

Have you felt baby moving today?

....

How many times?

....

How do you feel?

....
....
....
....
....
....
....

Forming a new habit takes about three weeks. So keep track of your progress. If you continuously have a Baby and Me Time for 21 days, you will have formed a new neural pathway and it is now a habit. Well done!

RUTH OSHIKANLU

Planning My Baby's Birth

Your *birth plan* helps communicate your wishes to the midwives and doctors caring for you in labour. It informs them about your wishes for labour, childbirth and after baby is born. You could either write your birth plan on a blank piece of baby or write it directly into your hand held notes. If there are any issues not covered in your birth plan then discuss them with your midwife.

Remember that you need to be flexible, as things may not go according to plan. Therefore, you should always have back-up plans.

If you ever needed a backup plan, what would it look like?

Now, prepare Plan B.

Plan B

If things don't go as planned, what would I do?

....

....

....

....

....

....

....

....

....

....

....

....

....

....

....

TUNE IN TO YOUR BABY: APPENDIX

Plan C

If my Plan B fails, what else would I do?

RUTH OSHIKANLU

How Do I Feel About Becoming a Mum? – Motherhood Gains and Losses

Motherhood Gains: What would love about being a mum?

....
....
....
....
....
....
....
....
....

Motherhood Losses: What would I lose because I am a mum?

....
....
....
....
....
....
....
....
....

TUNE IN TO YOUR BABY: APPENDIX

Prepare To Enjoy Motherhood

What's going to be challenging about becoming a mum?

....
....
....
....
....
....
....
....
....
....

What's going to be great about becoming a mum?

....
....
....
....
....
....
....
....
....
....
....

My Day Now!

What does my 24-hour day currently look like?

Time	Activity

TUNE IN TO YOUR BABY: APPENDIX

My Day After Baby's Here!

What will my 24-hour day look like after baby is born?

Time	Activity

RUTH OSHIKANLU

Feel Your Baby's Journey in to the World

Your baby's journey to the world was a stressful one. Try to *step into your baby's shoes*. Imagine what it felt like for your baby as s/he navigated his/her way down the birth canal.

What kind of labour and birth did you have?

....
....

Considering the type of birth you had, what do you think your baby's journey may have felt like for him/her?

....
....
....
....
....
....
....
....
....

How do you feel about what your baby may have experienced?

....
....
....
....

What will you do about it?

....

TUNE IN TO YOUR BABY: APPENDIX

Mimic the Womb, Outside the Womb

Your baby was very comfortable inside your womb. Now that baby is outside the womb, life is very different. Baby would love to go back, but that can't happen. To aid baby's transition to life outside the womb, it is important to try to mimic the conditions of the womb for baby.

How will you try to re-create the conditions baby is used to?

....
....
....
....
....
....
....
....

Your Baby's Cues

When your baby wants to interact with you, s/he will use **approach cues**. S/he will look at you, reach towards you, smile at you, babble, and talk to you. His/her eyes are usually bright and wide. This is often a good time to talk, play, and feed your baby.

Can you identify your baby's approach cues?

....
....
....
....
....
....
....
....

TUNE IN TO YOUR BABY: APPENDIX

When your baby is tired, needs a break from you or is distressed, s/he will use **withdrawal cues**. Your baby will often turn or pull away, arch his/her back, whine or fuss, squirm or kick, cry or sometimes vomit. Your baby may need to stop eating, playing, or being held. Sometimes your baby may get bored of a certain activity and require a change from what is happening. Your baby may do this by looking away, turning his/her head away, yawning, having a dull looking expression on his/her face, or putting his/her hands up to his/her face. Often when baby needs a change of pace, s/he becomes restless or more active.

Can you identify your baby's withdrawal cues?

....

....

....

....

....

....

....

Your Baby's States

Throughout the day, your baby will move through different levels of sleepiness and wakefulness. These levels are called 'states'.

Can you record the number of times in one day that your baby enters a different state?

Baby's State	Starting from the left hand side, put a tick in the appropriate box every time you notice your baby in that state (✓)								
Deep sleep									
Light sleep									
Drowsy/Dozing									
Quiet alert									
Active alert									
Crying									

Contain Your Baby's Emotions

Parents can help contain their babies by helping them cope with anxiety and emotions so they are not overwhelmed or disabled by the intensity of their feelings. A mum can do this by *stepping into baby's shoes* and imagining what her baby is feeling but not by taking his problem on.

What do you think about when your baby is crying?

....
....
....
....
....
....
....

How do you feel when your baby is crying?

....
....
....
....
....
....
....

What do you do when your baby is crying?

....
....
....
....
....
....
....

TUNE IN TO YOUR BABY: APPENDIX

Are you able to help soothe your baby without taking his pain on?

....
....
....
....

If you are able to do this, then you are being a *container* for your baby. Keep practising! In time, you will get better at doing it.

Breast-feeding Your Baby – How is it going?

What do you like about breast-feeding?

....
....
....
....
....
....
....

What do you find challenging?

....
....
....
....
....
....
....

How are you going to resolve these challenges? Who can support you?

....
....
....
....
....

TUNE IN TO YOUR BABY: APPENDIX

How does breast-feeding your baby, make you feel?

RUTH OSHIKANLU

Love for You, Baby and Others

How do you show that you love yourself?

How do you show your baby that you love him/her?

TUNE IN TO YOUR BABY: APPENDIX

How do you show that you love your significant other(s)?

RUTH OSHIKANLU

Playing With Your Baby

How do you play with your baby?

....
....
....
....
....
....
....
....
....
....

What games does your baby like to play?

....
....
....
....
....
....
....
....

Try to find out about local playgroups and take your baby to these. He/She will enjoy them.

How Do I Feel About Being A Mum? – Motherhood Gains and Losses

Motherhood Gains: Things that I love about being a mum

....
....
....
....
....
....
....
....
....
....

Motherhood Losses: Things that I have lost because I am a mum

....
....
....
....
....
....
....
....
....
....

RUTH OSHIKANLU

How Does It Feel To Be a Mum?

What's great about being a mum?

What is challenging about being a mum?

TUNE IN TO YOUR BABY: APPENDIX

How can you make it better?

RUTH OSHIKANLU

Celebrate Motherhood!
It's All About Learning and Growing.

Ask yourself the following questions every week:

What have I learned about myself during the past week?

....
....
....
....
....
....
....
....
....
....

What have I learned about my baby during the past week?

....
....
....
....
....
....
....
....
....
....

TUNE IN TO YOUR BABY: APPENDIX

What have I learned about my significant other(s) during the past week?

....
....
....
....
....
....
....
....
....
....

What have I learned about my role as a mum during the past week?

....
....
....
....
....
....
....
....
....
....
....
....

Where Are You in The Learning Circle?

The following questions can help you ascertain where you are in the learning circle. As you gain more knowledge and learn more skills as a parent, your confidence in parenting will grow. Keeping a record of skills acquired can boost your confidence when you need to learn a new skill. When you're learning a new skill, remember that you were once at level one for every other skill that you mastered. So persist in the learning process until the new skill is mastered.

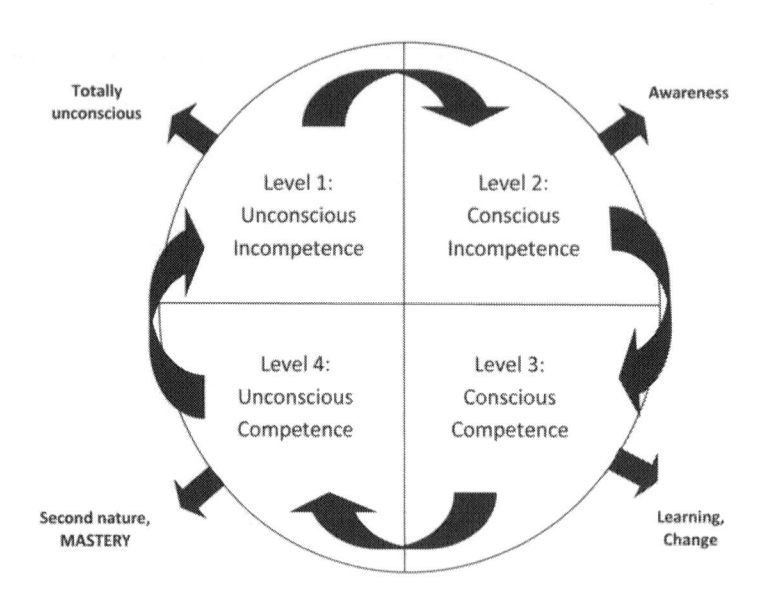

```
                    Totally                                    Awareness
                 unconscious

                          Level 1:              Level 2:
                        Unconscious            Conscious
                        Incompetence         Incompetence

                          Level 4:              Level 3:
                        Unconscious            Conscious
                        Competence            Competence

                 Second nature,                               Learning,
                   MASTERY                                     Change
```

The Circle of Learning

What skill are you trying to learn?

....

....

Do you feel you have enough information about the skill you are trying to learn?

....

TUNE IN TO YOUR BABY: APPENDIX

If not, what information do you require?
....
....

Who can help you get it?
....
....

Do you feel competent?
....

Do you feel confident?
....

Are you conscious about it?
....

Any other insights:
....
....
....

Making Adult Decisions - Weighing Up the Pros and Cons

Having choices is a good thing as it is empowering. However, making choices can bring with it huge responsibilities and can lead to indecision. When you have only one option, it is easy to choose because there is no decision required. When the options are many, decision making can be challenging. Whenever you have a decision to make and you are unsure what to do, the decision tool below can be useful.

Here are two examples of how to use the decision tool for making choices about feeding and childcare.

Choice of Feeding

	Breast-feeding	Bottle feeding
Pros		
Cons		

Choice of Childcare

	Nanny	Child-minder	Nursery
Pros			
Cons			

This decision tool can assist you in the decision-making process in almost any area where you have more than one option. All you have to do is to make columns out of the number of options you have and to list the pros and cons under each option/column.

RUTH OSHIKANLU

My Special Baby:

_____
(insert your baby's name)

What is special about _____? (insert your baby's name)

....
....
....
....
....
....
....
....
....
....

How does _____ being special make you feel?

....
....
....
....

Do you let _____ know?

....

Make it a habit to tell your baby every day, how special s/he is

TUNE IN TO YOUR BABY: APPENDIX

Could It Be Colic?

Remember the rule of 3 for Colic:

- Crying for more than 3 hours a day,
- For more than 3 days a week,
- For more than 3 weeks?

	How would you describe your baby's cry?	What signs did s/he show?	Time of day	Is it before or after feeds?	How long did your baby cry for?	What did you do to comfort your baby?	How did your baby respond?
Week 1							
Monday							
Tuesday							
Wednesday							
Thursday							
Friday							
Saturday							
Sunday							

If you observe any new symptoms, or baby's cry becomes weak and/or high-pitched, or baby's condition suddenly gets worse, then see your doctor who can refer you to a specialist.

Adapted from Unite/CPHVA Educational Supplement – Managing Colic (2012)

	How would you describe your baby's cry?	What signs did s/he show?	Time of day	Is it before or after feeds?	How long did your baby cry for?	What did you do to comfort your baby?	How did your baby respond?
Week 2							
Monday							
Tuesday							
Wednesday							
Thursday							
Friday							
Saturday							
Sunday							

If you observe any new symptoms, or baby's cry becomes weak and/or high-pitched, or baby's condition suddenly gets worse, then see your doctor who can refer you to a specialist.

Adapted from Unite/CPHVA Educational Supplement – Managing Colic (2012)

TUNE IN TO YOUR BABY: APPENDIX

	How would you describe your baby's cry?	What signs did s/he show?	Time of day	Is it before or after feeds?	How long did your baby cry for?	What did you do to comfort your baby?	How did your baby respond?
Week 3							
Monday							
Tuesday							
Wednesday							
Thursday							
Friday							
Saturday							
Sunday							

If you observe any new symptoms, or baby's cry becomes weak and/or high-pitched, or baby's condition suddenly gets worse, then see your doctor who can refer you to a specialist.

Adapted from Unite/CPHVA Educational Supplement – Managing Colic (2012)

RUTH OSHIKANLU

Teaching My Baby

What are you trying to teach _____ ?

For example, to sleep by him/herself, to eat solid food, etc.

....
....
....
....
....
....
....
....

How is it going?

....
....
....
....
....
....
....
....
....
....
....

TUNE IN TO YOUR BABY: APPENDIX

If it's taking longer than you expected for your baby to learn what you are trying to teach him/her, the tool below can be a useful exercise. It will also help you to learn delayed gratification.

	Giving up?	Persisting?
Pros		
Cons		

Find Your 20 Per Cent

Pareto's Principle suggests that just 20 per cent (one fifth) of what you do gives you 80 per cent (four fifths) of the results.

- What's the 20 per cent of what you do that makes the most difference in your life? i.e. What are your essentials, the non-negotiables, the must-dos?

....
....
....
....
....
....
....
....
....
....
....
....
....
....
....

Transfer the list to the table on the next page.

Now focus on doing this 20 per cent for 21 days. This is because it takes about three weeks to form a new habit.

TUNE IN TO YOUR BABY: APPENDIX

The 20 Per Cent That Makes the Most Difference	1	2	3	4	5	6	7	8	9	10	11	12	13	14	15	16	17	18	19	20	21

Having focused on your 20 per cent for 21 days, how do you feel?

....
....
....
....
....
....
....
....
....

Did it make a difference?

....

What difference did it make?

....
....
....
....
....
....
....
....
....

TUNE IN TO YOUR BABY: APPENDIX

My Daily Planner

Plan your day the night before. Imagine your day going the best way possible. Wake up in the morning and imagine it going the best way possible. As you complete activities, place a tick in the box. Observe how this makes you feel. At the end of each day, complete the *Review and Fix* section before planning your next day.

Time	20% Activities That Make a Difference	✓

Review and Fix
Successes (What did I love about today?)
Lessons (What did I learn today?)
Changes (If I had to relive today, what would I do differently?)

My Daily Planner

Plan your day the night before. Imagine your day going the best way possible. Wake up in the morning and imagine it going the best way possible. As you complete activities, place a tick in the box. Observe how this makes you feel. At the end of each day, complete the *Review and Fix* section before planning your next day.

Time	20% Activities That Make a Difference	✓

Review and Fix
Successes (What did I love about today?)
Lessons (What did I learn today?)
Changes (If I had to relive today, what would I do differently?)

My Daily Planner

Plan your day the night before. Imagine your day going the best way possible. Wake up in the morning and imagine it going the best way possible. As you complete activities, place a tick in the box. Observe how this makes you feel. At the end of each day, complete the *Review and Fix* section before planning your next day.

Time	20% Activities That Make a Difference	✓

Review and Fix

Successes (What did I love about today?)

Lessons (What did I learn today?)

Changes (If I had to relive today, what would I do differently?)

My Daily Planner

Plan your day the night before. Imagine your day going the best way possible. Wake up in the morning and imagine it going the best way possible. As you complete activities, place a tick in the box. Observe how this makes you feel. At the end of each day, complete the *Review and Fix* section before planning your next day.

Time	20% Activities That Make a Difference	✓

Review and Fix

Successes (What did I love about today?)

Lessons (What did I learn today?)

Changes (If I had to relive today, what would I do differently?)

TUNE IN TO YOUR BABY: APPENDIX

My Daily Planner

Plan your day the night before. Imagine your day going the best way possible. Wake up in the morning and imagine it going the best way possible. As you complete activities, place a tick in the box. Observe how this makes you feel. At the end of each day, complete the *Review and Fix* section before planning your next day.

Time	20% Activities That Make a Difference	✓

Review and Fix
Successes (What did I love about today?)
Lessons (What did I learn today?)
Changes (If I had to relive today, what would I do differently?)

My Daily Planner

Plan your day the night before. Imagine your day going the best way possible. Wake up in the morning and imagine it going the best way possible. As you complete activities, place a tick in the box. Observe how this makes you feel. At the end of each day, complete the *Review and Fix* section before planning your next day.

Time	20% Activities That Make a Difference	✓

Review and Fix

Successes (What did I love about today?)

Lessons (What did I learn today?)

Changes (If I had to relive today, what would I do differently?)

TUNE IN TO YOUR BABY: APPENDIX

My Daily Planner

Plan your day the night before. Imagine your day going the best way possible. Wake up in the morning and imagine it going the best way possible. As you complete activities, place a tick in the box. Observe how this makes you feel. At the end of each day, complete the *Review and Fix* section before planning your next day.

Time	20% Activities That Make a Difference	✓

Review and Fix

Successes (What did I love about today?)

Lessons (What did I learn today?)

Changes (If I had to relive today, what would I do differently?)

My Daily Planner

Plan your day the night before. Imagine your day going the best way possible. Wake up in the morning and imagine it going the best way possible. As you complete activities, place a tick in the box. Observe how this makes you feel. At the end of each day, complete the *Review and Fix* section before planning your next day.

Time	20% Activities That Make a Difference	✓

Review and Fix

Successes (What did I love about today?)

Lessons (What did I learn today?)

Changes (If I had to relive today, what would I do differently?)

TUNE IN TO YOUR BABY: APPENDIX

My Daily Planner

Plan your day the night before. Imagine your day going the best way possible. Wake up in the morning and imagine it going the best way possible. As you complete activities, place a tick in the box. Observe how this makes you feel. At the end of each day, complete the *Review and Fix* section before planning your next day.

Time	20% Activities That Make a Difference	✓

Review and Fix
Successes (What did I love about today?)
Lessons (What did I learn today?)
Changes (If I had to relive today, what would I do differently?)

My Daily Planner

Plan your day the night before. Imagine your day going the best way possible. Wake up in the morning and imagine it going the best way possible. As you complete activities, place a tick in the box. Observe how this makes you feel. At the end of each day, complete the *Review and Fix* section before planning your next day.

Time	20% Activities That Make a Difference	✓

Review and Fix
Successes (What did I love about today?)
Lessons (What did I learn today?)
Changes (If I had to relive today, what would I do differently?)

TUNE IN TO YOUR BABY: APPENDIX

My Daily Planner

Plan your day the night before. Imagine your day going the best way possible. Wake up in the morning and imagine it going the best way possible. As you complete activities, place a tick in the box. Observe how this makes you feel. At the end of each day, complete the *Review and Fix* section before planning your next day.

Time	20% Activities That Make a Difference	✓

Review and Fix
Successes (What did I love about today?)
Lessons (What did I learn today?)
Changes (If I had to relive today, what would I do differently?)

My Daily Planner

Plan your day the night before. Imagine your day going the best way possible. Wake up in the morning and imagine it going the best way possible. As you complete activities, place a tick in the box. Observe how this makes you feel. At the end of each day, complete the *Review and Fix* section before planning your next day.

Time	20% Activities That Make a Difference	✓

Review and Fix
Successes (What did I love about today?)
Lessons (What did I learn today?)
Changes (If I had to relive today, what would I do differently?)

TUNE IN TO YOUR BABY: APPENDIX

My Daily Planner

Plan your day the night before. Imagine your day going the best way possible. Wake up in the morning and imagine it going the best way possible. As you complete activities, place a tick in the box. Observe how this makes you feel. At the end of each day, complete the *Review and Fix* section before planning your next day.

Time	20% Activities That Make a Difference	✓

Review and Fix
Successes (What did I love about today?)
Lessons (What did I learn today?)
Changes (If I had to relive today, what would I do differently?)

My Daily Planner

Plan your day the night before. Imagine your day going the best way possible. Wake up in the morning and imagine it going the best way possible. As you complete activities, place a tick in the box. Observe how this makes you feel. At the end of each day, complete the *Review and Fix* section before planning your next day.

Time	20% Activities That Make a Difference	✓

Review and Fix

Successes (What did I love about today?)

Lessons (What did I learn today?)

Changes (If I had to relive today, what would I do differently?)

TUNE IN TO YOUR BABY: APPENDIX

My Daily Planner

Plan your day the night before. Imagine your day going the best way possible. Wake up in the morning and imagine it going the best way possible. As you complete activities, place a tick in the box. Observe how this makes you feel. At the end of each day, complete the *Review and Fix* section before planning your next day.

Time	20% Activities That Make a Difference	✓

Review and Fix

Successes (What did I love about today?)

Lessons (What did I learn today?)

Changes (If I had to relive today, what would I do differently?)

My Daily Planner

Plan your day the night before. Imagine your day going the best way possible. Wake up in the morning and imagine it going the best way possible. As you complete activities, place a tick in the box. Observe how this makes you feel. At the end of each day, complete the *Review and Fix* section before planning your next day.

Time	20% Activities That Make a Difference	✓

Review and Fix

Successes (What did I love about today?)

Lessons (What did I learn today?)

Changes (If I had to relive today, what would I do differently?)

TUNE IN TO YOUR BABY: APPENDIX

My Daily Planner

Plan your day the night before. Imagine your day going the best way possible. Wake up in the morning and imagine it going the best way possible. As you complete activities, place a tick in the box. Observe how this makes you feel. At the end of each day, complete the *Review and Fix* section before planning your next day.

Time	20% Activities That Make a Difference	✓

Review and Fix
Successes (What did I love about today?)
Lessons (What did I learn today?)
Changes (If I had to relive today, what would I do differently?)

My Daily Planner

Plan your day the night before. Imagine your day going the best way possible. Wake up in the morning and imagine it going the best way possible. As you complete activities, place a tick in the box. Observe how this makes you feel. At the end of each day, complete the *Review and Fix* section before planning your next day.

Time	20% Activities That Make a Difference	✓

Review and Fix

Successes (What did I love about today?)

Lessons (What did I learn today?)

Changes (If I had to relive today, what would I do differently?)

TUNE IN TO YOUR BABY: APPENDIX

My Daily Planner

Plan your day the night before. Imagine your day going the best way possible. Wake up in the morning and imagine it going the best way possible. As you complete activities, place a tick in the box. Observe how this makes you feel. At the end of each day, complete the *Review and Fix* section before planning your next day.

Time	20% Activities That Make a Difference	✓

Review and Fix
Successes (What did I love about today?)
Lessons (What did I learn today?)
Changes (If I had to relive today, what would I do differently?)

My Daily Planner

Plan your day the night before. Imagine your day going the best way possible. Wake up in the morning and imagine it going the best way possible. As you complete activities, place a tick in the box. Observe how this makes you feel. At the end of each day, complete the *Review and Fix* section before planning your next day.

Time	20% Activities That Make a Difference	✓

Review and Fix

Successes (What did I love about today?)

Lessons (What did I learn today?)

Changes (If I had to relive today, what would I do differently?)

TUNE IN TO YOUR BABY: APPENDIX

My Daily Planner

Plan your day the night before. Imagine your day going the best way possible. Wake up in the morning and imagine it going the best way possible. As you complete activities, place a tick in the box. Observe how this makes you feel. At the end of each day, complete the *Review and Fix* section before planning your next day.

Time	20% Activities That Make a Difference	✓

Review and Fix
Successes (What did I love about today?)
Lessons (What did I learn today?)
Changes (If I had to relive today, what would I do differently?)

A-69

Managing My Feelings

Each day, for one week, put an 'x' in the box that represents your highest feeling (towards the top) and your lowest feeling (towards the bottom).

How do I feel?	Mon	Tues	Wed	Thurs	Fri	Sat	Sun
Balanced							
Happy							
Content							
Anxious							
Hopeless							
Helpless							
Guilty							
Afraid							
Sad							
Tearful							
Depressed *							
Angry *							
Wanting to hurt myself *							
Wanting to hurt others *							
Suicidal *							
Other							

* If you experience any of these feelings then please read the section entitled **Important Notice**.

What brings you down?

....

....

....

....

TUNE IN TO YOUR BABY: APPENDIX

What lifts you up?
....
....
....
....

Every day, what helps your feelings become balanced, happy or contented?
....
....
....
....

What do you think you can do to keep your feelings balanced?
....
....
....
....

If you require help managing your feelings, where and when will you seek it?
....
....

Breaking My Thinking Pattern

What do I regularly think about myself?
....
....
....
....
....

Is it serving me? Does the way I think make me feel good or bad?
....
....
....
....
....

Is there a pattern to what I think about myself?
....
....
....
....
....

How often does this pattern occur?
....
....
....

TUNE IN TO YOUR BABY: APPENDIX

What happens before the pattern starts?
....
....
....
....
....

What causes it to increase my good feelings?
....
....
....
....
....
....

What causes it to decrease my good feelings?
....
....
....
....
....
....
....
....

I'm Going Back to Work – Plan For Success!

Now that you have decided that you are going back to work, here are some things you may need to consider:

What have you decided about feeding your baby?

....
....
....
....

How do you feel about this?

....
....
....
....

Childcare: what options do you have: Use the pros and cons of Choice of Childcare under *Making Adult Decisions - Weighing up the Pros and Cons*

....
....
....
....
....
....

Who is going to do the housework?

....
....

TUNE IN TO YOUR BABY: APPENDIX

If you don't have a partner. Who can help you?
....
....
....
....
....

How would they help you?
....
....
....

Do you require flexible working arrangements?
....

If so, what?
....
....
....
....
....

Have you enlisted your employer's support?
....
....
....
....

Why the Guilt?

Do you feel guilty about something?

If so, what makes you feel guilty?

....
....
....
....

Do you feel guilty about something that is happening now, or something that happened in the past?

....
....

If you feel guilty about something that's happening now, then remember that you are very powerful and can change what's happening now and create a different future.

But if you feel guilty about something that happened in the past, then remember that you can't change your past. However, you can change how you FEEL about the past.

Why do you feel guilty?

....
....
....
....

Are the reasons valid? If so, give evidence.

....
....
....

TUNE IN TO YOUR BABY: APPENDIX

....
....
....
....
....
....
....

Can you do anything different so that you can feel less guilty?

....

What can you do?

....
....
....
....
....
....
....
....
....
....

Now do it!

But go easy on yourself if you don't get the results you expect straight away. As you strive to make it a habit, you will get better at it.

Home and Work Swap

There are skills that you possess and employ at work that could be transferable to use at home and vice versa. List these skills below.

What home skills are you taking to work?	What work skills are you bringing home?

Why not try them in the opposite context and evaluate their benefit?

How have you benefitted from transferring these skills?

....
....
....
....

TUNE IN TO YOUR BABY: APPENDIX

More Loving, Playing and Learning

Why do you love _____? (Insert baby's name)

....
....
....
....

How do you let _____ know that you love him/her?

....
....
....
....
....
....
....
....

How does _____ respond?

....
....
....

How does this make you feel?

....
....
....

....
....
....
....
....

When do you play with _____?

....
....
....
....

What games does _____ like to play?

....
....
....
....
....
....
....
....
....
....
....

TUNE IN TO YOUR BABY: APPENDIX

How Much Sleep Does My Toddler Get?

Toddlers need more sleep than a child or adult, but less than a baby. An 18-month-old toddler needs about 13½ hours sleep daily, but may still have a nap of about two hours in the day. By the time they are two years of age, they may have a shorter nap in the day but will still sleep for almost 12 hours at night. By three, they will have an even shorter day nap (about an hour long) but will still sleep for almost twelve hours at night. However, this is a rough guide as each child is different. If you having problems with your toddler's sleep, keep a diary of their sleep pattern so that you can discuss it with your health visitor.

Time / Day of the Week	Time of Daytime Nap	Time Toddler Awakes	Time Bedtime Routine Starts	Time Toddler is Put into Bed	Time Toddler Goes to Sleep	Time Toddler Awakes	Total Number of Hours That Toddler is Asleep

My Toddler's Food Diary

Over a 24-hour period, your toddler should be offered three meals, two or three snacks and six to eight small cups of fluid. Offer your toddler a healthy, balanced diet. For example:

- At every meal, your toddler should be offered starchy foods (such as rice, potato, breads, pasta), fruits, and vegetables.

- Once or twice a day, offer him/her foods high in iron and protein (such as meats, chicken, fish, pulses like beans or lentils).

- Offer foods high in calcium like milk, cheese and yoghurt about three times daily. Limit the amount of milk your toddler drinks to about 360mls (12 fluid ounces). This can be divided into three portions of 120mls (4 fluid ounces). If your toddler is still thirsty offer him/her water, as giving too much milk can reduce his/her appetite. There is also no need for *growing up milk*, if your toddler is eating a healthy diet.

- If your toddler is fussy, you can supplement his/her diet with multivitamin drops or syrup.

If you are worried about his/her nutrition, you may want to keep a diary of his/her intake so that you can discuss this with your health visitor. Here's an example.

Day of the Week	Meal + Fluids	Snack + Fluids	Meal + Fluids	Snack + Fluids	Meal + Fluids	Snack + Fluids	Milk (Max.360mls)

TUNE IN TO YOUR BABY: APPENDIX

Planning for Tantrums

When does my toddler have tantrums?
....
....
....
....

Where does my toddler have tantrums?
....
....
....
....

What happens before, during and after my toddler has tantrums?
....
....
....
....
....
....
....
....
....
....
....

What can I do to prevent them from happening?

....
....
....
....
....
....
....
....
....
....
....

What can I do to manage them?

....
....
....
....
....
....
....
....
....
....
....

My Toddler Does Not Like the Potty

If despite all that you do your toddler refuses to use the potty, you may want to talk to him/her to find out why. Be empathic and support him/her when s/he tells you the reason why. Use a reward system just for potty training. Leave it where the potty is. Whenever your toddler uses the potty, give him/her verbal praise and put a star or reward sticker on a *reward chart*. If your toddler does have an accident, encourage him/her to assist you in cleaning up. In that way, they will learn in a loving way, that there are consequences for their behaviour. It may be useful to keep a diary, as some resistance to use the potty may be caused by your reaction, especially if your child is not using the potty, or is having accidents. Your reaction often reinforces their behaviour, instead of changing it. Keeping a diary will also help you if you need to discuss the issue with your health visitor.

Day / Time	Accidental soiling	What did your toddler do?	How did I respond?	Accidental soiling	What did your toddler do?	How did I respond?

Teaching My Toddler

What are you trying to teach _____?

For example, to sleep by him/herself, to eat new foods, etc.

....
....
....
....
....
....
....
....

How is it going?

....
....
....
....
....
....
....
....
....

TUNE IN TO YOUR BABY: APPENDIX

The following tool can be a useful exercise if it's taking longer than you expected for your toddler to learn what you are trying to teach him/her. It will also help you learn to delay your gratification.

	Giving up?	**Persisting?**
Pros		
Cons		

A-87

Playing With My Toddler

How do you play with your toddler?

....
....
....
....
....
....
....
....

What games does your toddler like to play?

....
....
....
....
....
....
....
....
....
....
....
....
....

TUNE IN TO YOUR BABY: APPENDIX

Positive Talk

It is important to avoid negative statements, as your toddler's brain doesn't understand them. Therefore, turn negative statements into positive ones. Here are a few examples:

Negative statement	**Positive statement**
Don't throw your toy.	Put your toy down.
Don't touch the television.	Move away from the television. Come and sit next to me.
No, don't do that!	State your child's name and tell them what it is you want them to do.

Now turn some of your previous negative statements into more positive ones.

Negative statement
....
Positive statement
....

Negative statement
....
Positive statement
....

Negative statement
....

Positive statement

....

Negative statement

....

Positive statement

....

Negative statement

....

Positive statement

....

Negative statement

....

Positive statement

....

Negative statement

....

Positive statement

....

Negative statement

....

Positive statement

....

TUNE IN TO YOUR BABY: APPENDIX

What is My Choice of Parenting Style?

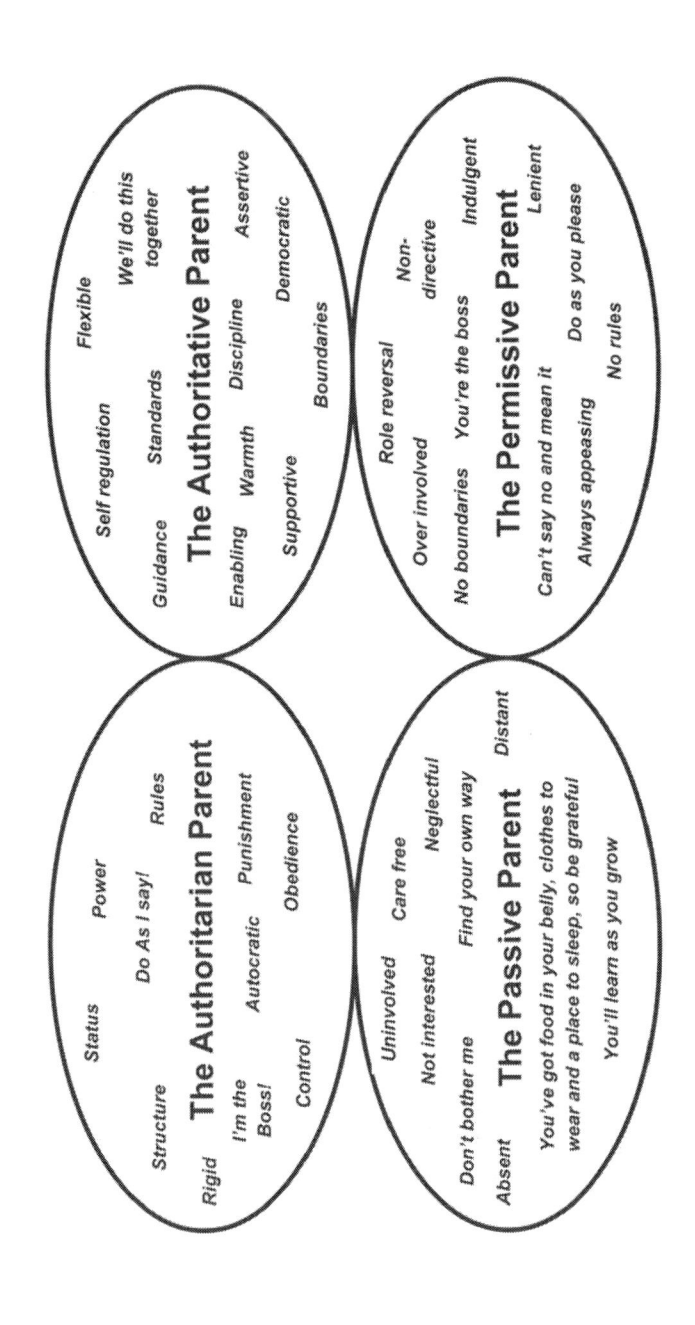

The Authoritative Parent
Flexible
We'll do this together
Self regulation
Assertive
Standards
Discipline
Democratic
Guidance
Warmth
Boundaries
Enabling
Supportive

The Permissive Parent
Non-directive
Indulgent
Lenient
Role reversal
You're the boss
Do as you please
Over involved
No boundaries
Can't say no and mean it
No rules
Always appeasing

The Authoritarian Parent
Power
Rules
Status
Do As I say!
Punishment
Autocratic
Obedience
Structure
I'm the Boss!
Control
Rigid

The Passive Parent
Distant
Care free
Neglectful
Uninvolved
Find your own way
Not interested
Don't bother me
You've got food in your belly, clothes to wear and a place to sleep, so be grateful
Absent
You'll learn as you grow

Parenting Styles

A-91

RUTH OSHIKANLU

My Special Toddler

_____
(insert your baby's name)

What is special about _____? (Insert your baby's name)

....
....
....
....
....
....
....
....
....
....

How does _____ being special make you feel?

....
....
....

Do you let _____ know?

....

Make it a habit to tell your baby, every day, how special s/he is.

Love For Yourself, Toddler and Others

How do you show that you love yourself?

....
....
....
....
....
....
....
....
....
....
....
....
....
....
....

How do you show your toddler that you love him/her?

....
....
....
....
....
....
....

How do you show that you love your significant other(s)?

Printed in Great Britain
by Amazon.co.uk, Ltd.,
Marston Gate.